THROMBOLYSIS: THE DAWN OF A NEW ERA?

THROMBOLYSIS: THE DAWN OF A NEW ERA?

Edited by P Sleight, University of Oxford, UK
and D A Chamberlain, Royal Sussex County Hospital, UK

IBC Technical Services Ltd

First published in Great Britain in 1990 by IBC Technical Services Ltd, Bath House (3rd Floor), 56 Holborn Viaduct, London EC1A 2EX.

British Library Cataloguing in Publication Data
Thrombolysis.
1. Man. Thrombolysis.
I. Sleight, Peter II. Chamberlain, D. A.
616.135

ISBN 1–85271–098–5

Typeset by Selectmove Ltd London
Printed and bound in Great Britain by Cotswold Group

Contents

FOREWORD

This timely and up to date book contains chapters by most of the leading authorities (both from industry and academe) on this exciting and fast moving field. It deals not only with presently available thrombolytics but also with the next generation of these, together with present and future adjuvant strategies.

It begins with an account of the early work with streptokinase by Dr Sol Sherry, who played such a large part in the clinical development of this agent. Sadly, its now proven benefit in myocardial infarction was not generally recognised until some 30 years after it was first used clinically. The large trials, GISSI-I and ISIS 2, which finally demonstrated its ability to reduce early mortality, themselves depended on a combination of factors. First and most compelling was the visualisation of coronary clot lysis by angiography by the pioneering work of Chazov in the Soviet Union and Rentrop in Germany. Next came the work of Schroder and his colleagues in Berlin in the development of the modern high dose intravenous infusion of streptokinase over one hour or less. After this the meta analysis by Yusuf *et al.* of all the available evidence on thrombolysis by streptokinase suggested that this treatment, then virtually abandoned, would reduce mortality by 20–25%.

Chapters then follow on the biology, pharmacology and clinical use of the four main agents currently in clinical use, namely streptokinase (Behringwerke-Hoechst), anistreplase (APSAC, SmithKline-Beecham), tissue Plasminogen activator (Alteplase – Genentech, Duteplase – Burroughs Wellcome), together with the latest arrival, pro-urokinase. The ASSET trial of Genentech t-PA and the AIMS study of anistreplase are discussed. Two chapters follow on the two recombinant tissue plasminogen activator agents – the single chain alteplase (Genentech, Dr Elliott Grossbard) and the Wellcome compound, Duteplase double-chain rt-PA (Dr Alastair Malcolm).

Two other important chapters are on the treatment of myocardial infarction by pre-hospital thrombolysis (Professor Jean-Pierre Boissel) and the role of thrombolysis in unstable angina (Professor Mirielle Brochier).

The important subject of adjuvant therapy, particularly the exciting new work on anti-thrombotic pathways and thromboxane receptor antagonists is dealt with by Dr E F Smith from Philadelphia. Dr E Fritsch outlines the development of mutants of rt-PA – the so-called second generation rt-PA (Genetics Institute, Cambridge, MA). Finally, who better than Professor Desire Collen from Leuven, the father of recombinant tissue plasminogen activator, to review the whole field and particularly point out the available information on second and third generation agents, particularly genetically engineered mutants of the original rt-PA.

The book is aimed primarily at those physicians and CCU nurses involved in acute myocardial infarction but makes fascinating reading for general physicians and anyone interested in the use of modern molecular biological techniques married to a common disease – the subject of great competition amongst the many pharmaceutical physicians and researchers who will read this book.

P SLEIGHT
D A CHAMBERLAIN

Chapter 1

OVERVIEW OF CURRENT THROMBOLYTIC AGENTS

Sol Sherry

Temple University, Philadelphia, PA, USA

Introduction

In the absence of contraindications, thrombolytic therapy is now considered as the desirable form of therapy for the immediate treatment of an acute myocardial infarction; also it has provided the incentive and spurred the development and clinical evaluation of newer thrombolytic agents. A remarkable amount of information has accumulated in the past few years with a growth rate that is still accelerating. This is indicative of a dynamic and evolving field of therapy where basic and applied concepts continue to change, and where observations made are no longer consistent with preconceived notions. The following is an attempt to integrate current information into a conceptual framework and to provide a basis for a comparative evaluation of the different thrombolytic agents.

Considering the need to limit the bibliography, the reader is encouraged to consult a number of recent review articles, [1–3] published proceedings of symposia[4–6] and monographs[7–10] which provide the basis for most of the statements made along with substantiating references.

Thrombolytic Agents and their Mechanisms of Action

There are six thrombolytic agents currently being used or evaluated for the immediate treatment of acute transmural myocardial infarction: streptokinase (SK), anisoylated plasminogen-streptokinase activator complex (APSAC), urokinase (UK), recombinant prourokinase (r proUK or r scu-PA), recombinant single stranded tissue-type plasminogen activator (rt-PA, one chain) and recombinant double stranded tissue-type plasminogen activator (rt-PA, 2 chain). As shown in Figure 1, all act directly or indirectly to activate plasminogen, the precursor of a native proteolytic enzyme system present in biological fluids and also bound to various surfaces (fibrin, platelets, interplatelet matrix, endothelial cells, etc.). Activation involves the splitting of the arg_{560}–val_{561} bond in plasminogen which exposes the serine protease enzyme center of plasmin. Plasmin is a nonspecific proteolytic enzyme which derives its special fibrinolytic properties by: a) the binding of plasminogen to fibrin during clotting, and b) the binding of the native activator t-PA to fibrin in close proximity to plasminogen following its release locally from endothelial cells. As a result, plasmin formation is facilitated on the fibrin surface and is independent of the various checks and balances governing and regulating plasminogen activation in the systemic circulation. To achieve fibrinolysis for therapeutic purposes, pharmacologic doses of plasminogen activators are administered systemically with the aim of utilizing and highly energizing the native mechanism but at the expense of systemic effects not observed under localized physiological conditions.

Of the various thrombolytic agents, SK, a bacterial protein, works by immediately combining with plasminogen on 1:1 molecular basis to form a plasminogen-streptokinase activator complex which has both binding properties for fibrin by virtue of its plasminogen moiety and an enzyme center capable of rapidly converting plasminogen to plasmin. APSAC is the plasminogen-streptokinase activator complex whose enzyme center has been inactivated by anisoylation. Upon administration, the compound binds to fibrin before significant and progressive

Figure 1 *Various thrombolytic agents currently in an advanced stage of clinical evaluation. All directly or indirectly act as activators of plasminogen (plasminogen activators) and owe their thrombolytic properties to the activation of fibrin-bound plasminogen. (Plg = plasminogen.)*

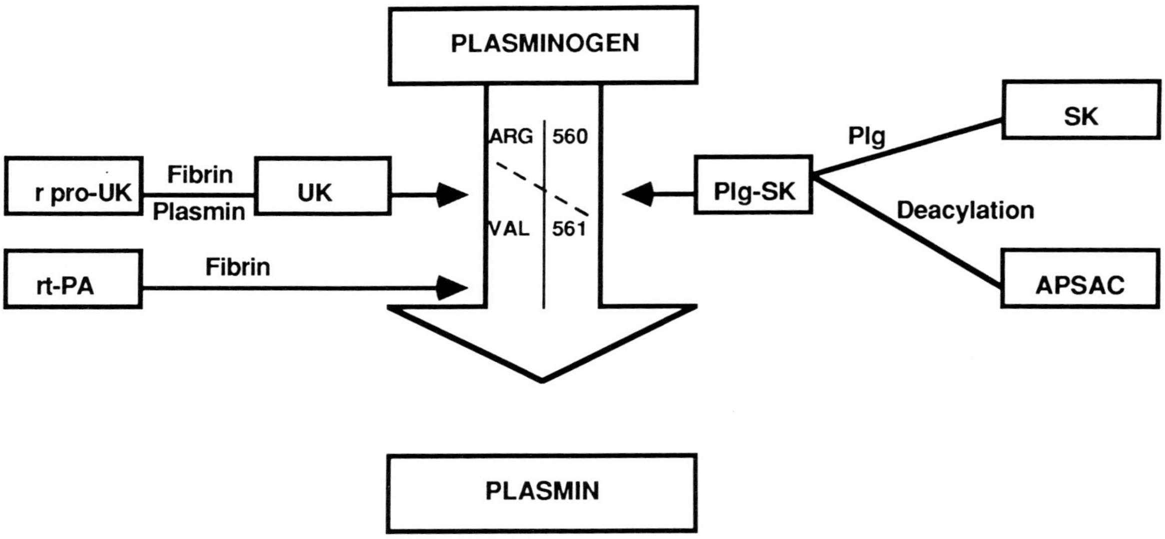

deacylation takes place; deacylation then liberates the active activator complex both on the fibrin surface and in plasma. As a consequence, there is more fibrin binding and more gradual release of the activator complex (extended pharmacokinetics) than observed with SK.

UK, a protein either isolated from urine or made by fetal human kidney cells in tissue culture, is a direct activator of plasminogen. Its single chain parent protein, prourokinase, is also made in tissue culture, but when made by genetic engineering, its production is by a bacterial cell. Native or recombinant proUK acts primarily on the fibrin surface. Though unlike t-PA it does not bind to fibrin; in the presence of trace amounts of plasmin it is converted to urokinase. The single and double chain t-PA's are also made by a recombinant DNA technique; a Chinese hamster ovary cell line has been utilized for yielding the most commonly employed forms of this human-type activator. The differences in molecular structure of the two forms are primarily due to the method of production (roller bottle or suspension culture). Both forms bind strongly to fibrin and the latter acts as a co-factor in the activation of plasminogen. It is believed that the single chain form is converted to the double chain form on the fibrin surface. While there are some *in vivo* differences in the action of these two forms, at current dosage recommendations they are reasonably similar in their effects[11] and consequently, for this discussion, they will be treated as one entity.

Because of its strong fibrin-binding properties, rt-PA is termed fibrin selective.* ProUK is also fibrin selective but for reasons other than fibrin-binding. The others, SK, APSAC and UK, are

*A more accurate designation for r t-PA would be surface selective since it binds to all surfaces (platelet, endothelial cell, etc.) where plasminogen is bound and acts preferentially in plasminogen activation on such surfaces. Physiologically the immediate role of t-PA appears to be one of limiting excessive hemostasis and thrombus growth; its action in thrombus resolution is a slower one.

referred to as non-fibrin selective. However all of the thrombolytic agents have preference for the activation of fibrin-bound plasminogen over that of plasma plasminogen,[12] and in currently recommended dosages, probably are fairly comparable in the speed and extent of activation of fibrin-bound plasminogen. However there are two differences. First, agents like rt-PA which bind to fibrin independent of the latter's binding sites for plasminogen continue to act on fibrin even after the circulating agent has been inactivated or cleared from the plasma. Consequently, they are more apt to dissolve aging or more lysis resistant fibrin as compared to the non-binding agents. (Resistance to lysis of fibrin increases with time after fibrin formation *in vivo* due to polymer crosslinking, clot retraction and compaction.) Second, the fibrin selective agents like rt-PA and proUK do not activate plasma plasminogen as well as the non-fibrin selective agents, for it is the speed and extent of *plasma* plasminogen activation which determines the degree of plasma proteolysis, i.e. the severity of fibrinogenolysis, the degradation of Factors V and VIII, the quantity of breakdown products and the resulting coagulation defect. A comparison of the speed and extent of plasma plasminogen activation with currently recommended regimens of the various agents is SK = APSAC > UK > r proUK = rt-PA.

Comparative Pharmacologic Features

A summary of several comparative pharmacologic features of the various thrombolytic preparations as infused intravenously in currently recommended regimens for the treatment of acute myocardial infarction is shown in Table 1. Preparations of SK and APSAC are known to be antigenic; UK is not, nor is it likely that rt-PA or r proUK will be antigenic (the possibility remains of some antigens from the nonhuman cell sources). The fibrin selective agents have a significantly shorter half-life as compared to the non-fibrin selective agents; APSAC, as chemically designed, has the longest half-life. All of the agents lyse hemostatic plugs as effectively as they do a thrombus since both are stabilized by a fibrin mesh; however those agents which are more capable of dissolving aging thrombi will be more effective in lysing older hemostatic plugs. The fibrinogenolytic response to thrombolytic therapy in patients is variable regardless of the agent used; therefore the comparison shown in Table 1 refers to the average reaction. Fibrinogenolysis with SK therapy is very extensive; all the native fibrinogen is degraded into a number of fibrinogen fragments (X, Y, D, E). Fragment X, a thrombin coagulable but slowly polymerizing protein molecule, accounts for the clottability of the blood which is slow and of poor tensile strength. The extent of fibrinogenolysis with APSAC is similar to that described for SK, both of which are somewhat greater than that associated with UK therapy. More modest fibrinogenolysis is observed during therapy with the fibrin selective agents regimens but, even here, most of the native fibrinogen is degraded.[13] However since the extent of fibrinogenolysis is more limited, better clottability is maintained due in great part to higher concentrations of clottable protein (fragment X and its partially degraded precursors). Nevertheless recovery, as with the non-fibrin selective agents is delayed since return to a normal coagulation mechanism is dependent on relatively slow rates of new fibrinogen synthesis and clearance of breakdown products from the circulation; on average, a full recovery requires 36–48 hours following termination of the therapy.

Factors to be Considered in Clinical Evaluation

The primary objective of thrombolytic therapy for the treatment of an acute evolving myocardial infarction is to limit irreversible damage to heart muscle by stopping the progression of the infarct and to reduce mortality associated with the event.

Table 1 *Comparative pharmacologic features in vivo of various thrombolytic preparations as used in acute MI*

Feature	*SK*	*APSAC*	*UK*	*rt-PA*	*r ProUK*
Antigenicity	Yes	Yes	No	No(?)	No(?)
Half-life (min.)	23	90	16	5	7
Specificity: Clot vs. hemostatic plug	None	None	None	None	None
Fibrinogenolysis (++++ = most extensive)	++++	++++	+++	++	++

Myocardial Salvage. Since the infarction of tissue from a sustained ischemic event starts early, progresses rapidly and is essentially completed within 4 hours, little benefit can be expected when the treatment is started late. Consequently, a comparative evaluation of the efficacy of the various thrombolytic agents as far as myocardial salvage is concerned needs to be restricted to that period when practical clinical benefit is still possible, i.e., up to 4 hours from symptom onset and preferably earlier. Further, the evaluation and comparison reflects a combination of all the possible benefits (incidence of reperfusion within this time frame, improvement in flow rates, reduction in cardiac strain), and all of the possible debits (incidence of serious bleeding complications, early reocclusion and other adverse reactions) in arriving at a risk/benefit and cost/benefit ratio for the particular agent.

Mortality Reduction. It is becoming evident that mortality reduction can still be achieved by thrombolytic therapy even beyond the four-hour period when significant myocardial salvage is likely to be accomplished.[14] In retrospect, this should have been suspected on the basis of the various trials conducted during the 1960s and 70s with intravenously administered streptokinase; randomization in these trials covered the period from 4 to 24 hours after the onset of symptom onset, nevertheless meta analysis [15,16] revealed a reduction of mortality of approximately 20%. Direct documentation of this dissociation between significant myocardial salvage and mortality reduction was noted first in the Western Washington trial of intracoronary streptokinase[17] where the mean time to randomization was 4.6 hours; the treatment group did not show any improvement in myocardial function yet there was a significant reduction in mortality. The recent AIMS study[18] where mortality reduction following intravenously administered APSAC was similar for patients entered 0–4 hours and 4–6 hours after the onset of symptoms, and the ISIS-2 study[14] where patients administered streptokinase intravenously beyond 4 hours and up to 24 hours had a lowered death rate, have confirmed that significant reductions in mortality can be obtained by thrombolytic therapy well beyond the period of demonstrable improvement in myocardial function. The explanation for this mortality reduction when the therapy is administered late is still unclear. Kennedy *et al.*[19] attributed this to reperfusion and possibly the salvage of some subepicardial myocardium. Or it is possible that reperfusion removes accumulating toxic products that contribute to mortality? Another alternative explanation is that APSAC and streptokinase, by virtue of the extensive fibrinogenolysis and viscosity reduction they produce (see below), improve flow rates, reduce afterload and cardiac strain. Forthcoming trials comparing t-PA and streptokinase on mortality rates both within the first 4 hours following symptom onset and for later periods of time could shed light on the possible mechanism(s) responsible for the overlapping of mortality reduction beyond the time frame of demonstrable myocardial salvage.

Table 2 *Comparative clinical pharmacologic features of various thrombolytic preparations as used in acute MI*

Feature	*SK*	*APSAC*	*UK*	*rt-PA*	*r proUK*
Incidence of patency at 90 min (%) (Rx 3 hrs)	60–65	65–70	60–70	65–75	60–70
Speed of reperfusion (minutes)	+++	++++	+++	++++	+++
Ease of administration	+++	++++	++	+	+++
Hemostatic effects:					
clotting defect	++++	++++	+++	++	++
platelet activation	++++	++++	0	++++	++
platelet aggregation	++	++	0	++++	?
Heparin need	no	no	no?	yes?	yes?
Bleeding incidence					
invaded sites	++++	++++	++++	++++	++++
non-invaded	+	+	+	+	+
Bleeding severity	++	?	?	++++	?
Rethrombosis (%)	10–15	5–10	5–10	15–25	?
Allergy	yes	yes	no	?	?
Expense	+	++–+++	++++	++–+	++++

0 (none) to ++++(greatest)
? sufficient information not yet available.

Comparison of Clinical Pharmacologic Features

A comparison of clinical pharmacologic features which accompanies currently recommended regimens of therapy with the various thrombolytic agents is shown in Table 2.

Patency and Speed of Reperfusion. When therapy is carried out within the first 3 hours following symptom onset, patency rates at the conclusion of therapy, or shortly thereafter, do not appear to be very different for the various agents nor are they very different in the speed at which their effects are evident though rt-PA appears to be faster than r proUK.

In the TIMI trial where therapy was begun 4.8 hours, on average, following symptom onset and observations made while t-PA was being infused (before rethrombosis) but not so for streptokinase (during rethrombosis), rt-PA was twice as effective as SK in reperfusing occluded vessels though there was no difference in clinical outcome[20] nor significant salvage of myocardium possible or observed.[21] However at the time of initiation of therapy in this study a fibrin-binding agent like rt-PA enjoys an advantage over SK in dissolving aged fibrin (see above). Further analysis of the data from the two studies[22,23] which allow for a comparison of the relative efficacy of rt-PA to SK (rt-PA/SK ratio) at different time intervals following symptom onset in patency or reperfusion rates, as shown in Figure 2, demonstrates that this superiority progressively disappears the earlier therapy is started after symptom onset. The data also suggest that within the first 2 hours of symptom onset the two agents are equally effective, nor is there a statistically significant difference between the agents when therapy is begun, on average, within the first 3.2 hours, i.e., within the time frame when meaningful myocardial salvage is

Figure 2 *Relative efficacy of intravenous rt-PA versus SK (rt-PA/SK ratio) in vessel reperfusion or patency as a function of average time to onset of therapy following onset of symptoms of acute myocardial infarction in comparative randomized trials.* ○, *TIMI phase I reperfusion data;*[22] ●, *European Cooperative Study Group patency data.*[23] *Equivalence projected to occur at 2 h.*

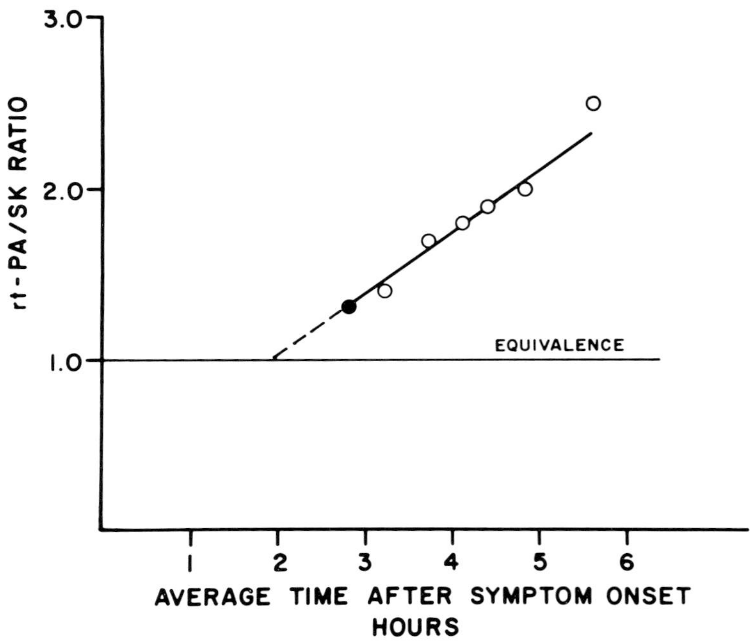

still possible. SK is not alone in being more effective on fresh fibrin than on aging fibrin; similar observations have been made in randomized trials with the other non-fibrin selective agents, UK[24] and APSAC.[25] The estimate in Table 2 of patency at 90 min of the infarct-related artery when therapy is begun within the first 3 hours of symptom onset is based on observations reported in various studies with SK, APSAC, UK, rt-PA, r proUK.

Since most of the controversy on patency rates has been with SK, the best data come from a randomized trial whose objective was restricted to its measurement. In the dose ranging study by Six[26] 189 patients were treated within 4 hours of symptom onset with a 1 hour infusion in a double-blind setting followed by angiographic evaluation at 2.8 hours on average following the onset of therapy. The patients treated with 0.2, and the more effective doses of 0.75, 1.5 or 3.0 million units, had patency rates of 38, 75, 60 and 82% respectively.

Patency data on urokinase in the German Activator Urokinase Study[24] which was a comparison between urokinase and t-PA in the treatment of acute myocardial infarction was 66%; this was not different from the 69% observed for rt-PA. Though unproven, the incidence of reperfusion is usually considered a more accurate estimate of the efficacy of clot dissolution than the patency incidence which is usually 10–15% higher because of the inclusion before therapy of subtotal occlusions. Nevertheless, sluggish flow around a subtotal thrombotic occlusion could just as well be responsible for precipitating an acute myocardial infarction as a totally obstructed vessel and, because of a larger area of thrombus exposed in a subtotal occlusion, it is more readily dissolved by the lytic process.

Even angiography while used as a gold standard for measuring the thrombolytic efficacy of an agent has its problems: it does not measure flow rates adequately[27] or the presence of distal run-off or the final end-point (repetitive opening and closing of occluded vessels during thrombolytic therapy is fairly common and the timing of the end-point has been an arbitrary one)—all of which are critical in determining myocardial salvage.

The absence of flow rates is a serious deterrent in the evaluation of the thrombolytic efficacy of an agent since flow rates will determine how quickly the anoxic event will be terminated, toxic products removed, and the likelihood of rethrombosis. In this regard, it is important to note that SK therapy, presumably because of the extensive fibrinogenolysis it produces, is associated with a significant reduction in plasma and, at low shear rates, in blood viscosity;[28,29] this counteracts the increased blood viscosity observed during acute infarction.[30] Since UK and APSAC therapy also produce extensive fibrinogenolysis, it is likely that similar viscosity changes will occur with the other non-fibrin selective agents. On the other hand, in the study of Jan *et al.*,[28] the milder fibrinogenolysis observed with rt-PA therapy was not associated with a significant fall in plasma and blood viscosity, nor is a reduction in viscosity likely to occur with r proUK therapy. Not only will a reduction in blood and plasma viscosity increase flow rates in the circulation of the infarct area but throughout the entire vascular tree as well; this could be expected to result in a reduction of afterload. Some evidence supporting a latter action already exists for SK[31] and may play a significant role in determining the clinical benefits associated with the therapy.

Ease of Administration. As shown in Table 2 there are differences in the ease of administration of the recommended regimens for the various thrombolytic agents. The 30-unit dose of APSAC is administered over a very brief period (2–5 minutes) and represents an advantage over the others; 1.5 million units of SK is infused over a period of up to one-hour;* 3 million units of UK (half as a loading dose) currently is being given over a 90-minute period; 100 mg rt-PA (60% in the first hour) is instilled over a 3-hour period; the dosage and duration of therapy with r proUK continues to undergo modification (most recently 60 mg has been given over a 60-minute period following a 20 mg bolus injection).

Systemic Hemostatic Defect. The severity of the clotting defect induced by each of the thrombolytic agents in currently recommended regimens mirrors the degree of fibrinogenolysis and is greatest for the non-fibrin selective agents as shown in Table 2. Less well recognized is that there is more to the hemostatic aberration than the hypocoagulable state; thrombolytic therapy is associated with platelet dysfunction. The ability of platelets to aggregate in response to many agonists (ADP, thrombin, epinephrine) depends on their ability to expose receptor sites on the platelet surface (the glycoprotein IIb/IIIa complex) for fibrinogen; the latter then provides the bond between apposing platelets. This bond becomes reinforced by the release of thrombospondin, a platelet specific protein, with a 'lectin-like' action and responsible for forming a glue-like intercellular matrix until further stabilized by the laying down of fibrin. Thus during thrombolytic therapy the ability of platelets to aggregate and form a stable mass is influenced by the availability of fibrinogen, exposure of the glycoprotein IIb/IIIa complex and the subsequent stability of the platelet aggregate; the first is more susceptible to the non-fibrin selective agents but the latter two probably are more susceptible to surface binding agents because of their advantage in activating plasminogens which are surface-bound (activation of platelet-bound plasminogen results initially in the exposure of the glycoprotein IIb/IIIa complex with enhanced platelet aggregatability, while activation of thrombospondin-bound plasminogen enhances platelet disaggregation). These induced defects in platelet function supplement the coagulation defect, and result in a more extensive systemic hemostatic aberration which enhances both the risk of bleeding and of rethrombosis.

Local Platelet Activation and Heightened Coagulability. Remarkably, while the systemic state during thrombolytic therapy is prohemorrhagic, the situation at the site of the local thrombotic

*SK is administered more slowly than APSAC since too rapid administration frequently is accompanied by a rapid drop in blood pressure postulated to be due to plasmin activation of prekallikrein and the release of bradykinin. Noteworthy is that in a recent study, the SK dose was administered over 30 minutes without problem[32] and, in another, 600,000 units was given as a bolus injection;[33] both reported favorable outcomes as to mortality when compared to the placebo group.

episode is prothrombotic.[34] This is due in part to significant elements of thrombogenicity (both platelet activation and heightened coagulability) produced by the therapy. Evidence for platelet activation *in vivo* is based on the demonstration of thromboxane release during and following thrombolytic therapy.[35,36] While direct comparison among agents has not been made, platelet activation probably is greatest with rt-PA (in the TIMI Phase I trial,[37] thrombocytopenia was more common in the r-tPA group), and appears to be least with urokinase.[38] Activation of clotting[39] and heightened coagulability locally at the site of the thrombotic event is due to the persistence of a thrombogenic stimulus at the thrombotic site and the transient conversion by plasmin of Factor V and, probably VIII, to activated forms (Va, VIIIa) before being more extensively degraded.[40] In this respect agents like rt-PA, which are administered during a more extended period of therapy and activate plasma plasminogen slowly and progressively, should have a more prolonged effect than observed during therapy with non-fibrin selective agents where plasmin formation and its inactivation is over with more rapidly.

Heparin Need. Heparin has been administered during therapy with rt-PA and r proUK with the aim of enhancing their action and reducing the incidence of rethrombosis. On the other hand, the extensive activation of plasma plasminogen which occurs during therapy with the non-fibrin selective agents produces a state of poor coagulability; consequently, heparin need not be administered simultaneously with these agents, and its administration, if deemed necessary, can be delayed until there is partial recovery from the induced hemostatic defect.

Whether heparin's antithrombotic properties exceed its contributions to heightened local thrombogenicity and systemic bleeding remains to be established (under evaluation in GISSI 2). Heparin's effectiveness as an anthrombotic agent before and after thrombolytic therapy can be questioned both on the basis of theoretical considerations and clinical observation for the following reasons: 1) heparin does not prevent platelet activation and, in the arterial tree, anticoagulants are not as effective in preventing thrombosis as are antiplatelet agents; 2) heparin (presumably the higher molecular weight forms) binds to platelets, activates them and can be responsible for platelet aggregation, platelet thrombosis and thrombocytopenia[41] with the latter also acting to increase the risk of bleeding; 3) heparin therapy augments the platelet activation of thrombolytic therapy;[42] 4) heparin activated antithrombin III, while capable of blocking thrombin action in blood, is incapable of inhibiting fibrin formation on the platelet surface[43] nor is it clear whether it can neutralize fibrin-bound thrombin; 5) high rates of rethrombosis during thrombolytic therapy cannot be prevented by simultaneous heparin administration.[44, 45]

Bleeding Complications. Fibrin selective agents, because of their milder effect on the coagulation mechanism were expected to have a lower incidence of bleeding complications. No evidence to support this assumption has been forthcoming. For all agents, severe bleeding, i.e. requiring transfusions, has been a frequent complication in the presence of recent invasive procedures; in the absence of the latter the incidence has been sharply reduced. Nevertheless there does appear to be a difference between rt-PA therapy and that observed with SK; rather than being safer, rt-PA therapy appears to be associated with greater transfusion requirements[37] and a higher incidence of intracerebral bleeding.[46, 47] The probable explanation is that agents which may be more efficacious in lysing fibrin, especially on older fibrin and are administered over a longer period of time, are more likely, by virtue of the dissolution of hemostatic plugs, to induce more serious bleeding.

In support of this view are the observations made in controlled trials. When invasive procedures are employed, bleeding has been frequent and occurs most often at such sites; when invasive procedures are avoided, the incidence of bleeding complications has been low. Also during clinical use, it is well recognized that vascular injury due either to recent surgery, trauma (including cardio-pulmonary resuscitation) or disease (stroke, peptic ulcer, etc.) are important risk factors for bleeding episodes. Furthermore, in controlled trials, the incidence of bleeding complications has shown little correlaion with the extent of fibrinogenolysis or of the 'lytic state' produced by a particular thrombolytic agent,[48, 49] and the incidence of bleeding complications between agents has shown little correlation with the extent of the fibrinogenolytic state they induce.[37, 50] That the coagulation defect attributable to thrombolytic therapy is an unlikely primary cause of a bleeding complication should have been suspected for, in the presence of an intact vascular system and a previously normal hemostatic mechanism, blood incoagulability produced by heparin or defibrinogenating therapy can be carried out with a relatively low risk of a hemorrhagic episode.

Rethrombosis. Many factors influence rethrombosis during and after thrombolytic therapy; in the last analysis it is the interplay between the presence of a local thrombogenic stimulus, the ability of the blood (platelets and the coagulation mechanism) to react to this stimulus, and the dynamics of blood flow. However, multiple factors may be involved in each of these variables.

That a thrombogenic stimulus persists after thrombolytic therapy is not unexpected. Lysis of the thrombus may re-expose the underlying lesion (crack, fissure, ulcer, etc.) in the atheromatous plaque originally responsible for the coronary thrombosis; or residual thrombus due to incomplete lysis, as is commonly present, will have thrombin bound to its surface[51] which serves as stimulus for platelet aggregation and new fibrin formation. In addition, as previously noted, thrombolytic therapy can increase the coagulability of blood and aggregatability of platelets, the latter being enhanced by heparin therapy. In some patients, heightened aggregation may also be due to the replacement of older platelets with more actively hemostatic younger ones This local prothrombotic state is offset in part by the extent of the induced coagulation defect. Therefore it is not surprising that the incidence of rethrombosis has been highest with rt-PA therapy;[22] its coagulation defect is more modest and there is more prolonged activation of platelets, and Factors V and VIII.

Two aspects of rethrombosis need to be emphasized since it is the major deterrent to successful thrombolytic therapy:

First is that the thrombus is in a dynamic state between two opposing forces: thrombus resolution, and new thrombus formation. Both are proceeding during thrombolytic therapy for the reasons previously cited. Thus the prevention of new thrombus formation during therapy could accelerate the speed of thrombus resolution, result in a higher patency rate and reduce the incidence of reocclusion. Originally it was believed that heparin would be useful for this purpose but standard heparin preparations have not been successful. However agents which inhibit platelet activation have been found to accomplish this role experimentally,[36, 52, 53] and their use probably accounts for the improved results obtained when aspirin was combined with streptokinase therapy in the ISIS-2 study[14].

Second, the beneficial results of the combined therapy group in ISIS-2 suggest that asymptomatic reocclusions also may occur following thrombolytic therapy and may be capable of increasing mortality; this implies that reports on reinfarction rates in various trials may underestimate the clinical problem.

Allergy. SK and APSAC, because of their antigenicity are not recommended for reuse for a period of 6 months, i.e., until the antibody level returns to the pretreatment concentration; otherwise the recommended dose is hardly likely to overcome the resistance to plasminogen activation.

Allergic reactions to SK and APSAC are also observed but the incidence is modest. Anaphylactoid reactions have occurred in 0.1 to 0.2% while rash, urticaria and hypotension have been observed in approximately 2.0 to 4.0%. The allergic reactions appear to be readily responsive to antihistamines and steroids, while the hypotensive episodes may require a dopamine infusion.

Expense. There is a wide range of cost of the various thrombolytic agents. Those produced by genetic engineering or tissue culture are very expensive. SK is the least expensive.

Table 3 *Comparative clinical results in randomized trials on myocardial salvage and mortality reduction with various thrombolytic preparations as used during therapy of acute myocardial infarction*

Clinical result	*SK*	*APSAC*	*UK*	*rt-PA*	*r proUK*
Myocardial salvage	yes	yes		yes	
Mortality reduction	yes	yes		yes	

Clinical Results

In the last analysis, only reductions in infarct size and mortality are of primary importance in comparing the clinical efficacy of different thrombolytic agents in currently recommended regimens. These benefits are not necessarily related to the incidence of reperfusion or patency rates alone or of other ancillary actions; the incidence of complications as they may result in permanent disability, death and hospital costs also enter into the risk/benefit and cost/benefit ratios for each drug.

In Table 3 is shown the present status of information in randomized trials on reduction of infarct size (usually implied through measurements of ventricular function at some time after the therapy when there is recovery of 'stunned' but still salvageable myocardium, and referred to as myocardial salvage) and mortality. The three trials comparing rt-PA with SK on myocardial function have shown little or no difference [21, 54, 55] nor has there been a difference when rt-PA has been compared with UK.[24] Nor are there any reported results as yet comparing one agent with another on mortality, though this is the object of the rt-PA versus SK comparison in GISSI-2, and the rt-PA, SK and APSAC comparison in ISIS-3. Consequently in Table 3, 'Yes' is noted where there has been evidence of a significant benefit and a blank space where appropriate data are not yet available. It is to be noted that myocardial salvage has been documented for SK[32, 56–60] and for r-tPA[47, 61–63] and recently for APSAC[64] but not as yet for the others. As for mortality reduction this has been well established for SK therapy both in terms of short- and long-term benefits,[14, 32, 57, 65, 66] for APSAC[18] and rt-PA.[47, 67]

Previous reference has been made to the results of the ISIS-2 study, the largest randomized trial of the effects of thrombolytic therapy on mortality. In this study over 17,000 patients were randomized to receive either streptokinase intravenously, 1.5 million units over 1 hour; aspirin 160 mg daily for 1 month; both; or neither. The mortality rate over the first 35-day period postinfarction was the primary endpoint. The objectives of the study were to determine: over what period of time during the first 24 hours following the onset of chest pain streptokinase therapy was still effective in reducing mortality; whether aspirin therapy started at a similar time interval could, by inhibiting platelet aggregation, reduce mortality; and whether the combination of thrombolytic and aspirin therapy would supplement each other in reducing mortality. The results were highly favorable for reduction of mortality either by streptokinase or aspirin when therapy was initiated at any point within the first 24 hours. This confirmed older studies with intravenously administered streptokinase as reviewed by Yusuf *et al.*[15] and Stampfer *et al.*[16], and is also consistent with and extends previous evidence supporting a reduction in the incidence of fatal and nonfatal myocardial infarction by aspirin therapy when initiated in patients within the first few weeks following a myocardial infarction[68]. The most impressive results were obtained with the combination therapy. One suspects that in the future, antiplatelet agents will replace heparin as the antithrombotic therapy of choice in the follow-up of patients who have received thrombolytic therapy.

APSAC also appears to be a very promising agent. In the AIMS trial,[18] which had to be terminated prematurely because of ethical reasons, APSAC reduced 30-day mortality by almost 48% when administered intravenously within the first 6 hours following the onset of symptoms. Furthermore, the reduction was similar in patients treated from 0 to 4 and 4 to 6 hours.

Since all of the agents are associated with a high patency rate following their administration within the first three hours following symptom onset (Table 2), it is highly likely that all will be associated with myocardial salvage and mortality reduction, and probably to a comparable degree, when administered early. Nevertheless data on the relative efficacy of agents in comparative trials are sorely needed; fortunately several such studies on myocardial salvage or mortality (GISSI-2) are already under way or will be started shortly (ISIS-3).

Fibrin Binding Vs. Non-Fibrin Binding

In the absence of comparative clinical data establishing greater benefit of one agent over another in reducing myocardial damage and mortality, current observations on thrombolytic therapy for acute myocardial infarction raise a serious question as to whether direct fibrin binding of a plasminogen activator provides any unusual or distinct advantage in thrombolytic therapy. Considering that all of the agents are active thrombolytically and that there are advantages and disadvantages to both fibrin and non-fibrin selective agents, as summarized in Table 4, it would appear, at present, that this aspect of drug action may not play a significant or key role in determining the clinical benefits of therapy[69].

Summary

All of the plasminogen activators which are in advanced stages of clinical evaluation, are capable of lysing most fresh thrombi and, when administered within the first few hours following

Table 4 *Relative advantages and disadvantages of 'fibrin-bound' (e.g. rt-PA) and 'non fibrin selective' (e.g. SK, APSAC, UK) thrombolytic agents as used in treatment of acute myocardial infarction*

'Fibrin-bound'	*'Non-fibrin selective'*
Advantages	
Extended action on fibrin surface	Induced anticoagulant state
Acts well on fresh and aging fibrin	Platelet aggregation impaired
Limited coagulation disturbance	Reduced blood and plasma viscosity
	Reduced afterload
	Short duration therapy
Disadvantages	
High rate of rethrombosis	Does not act well on aging fibrin
Longer period of therapy	Transient but extensive coagulation defect
Bleeding episodes more severe	
No reduction in afterload or in blood and plasma viscosity	
No evidence of greater clinical benefit	

the onset of an acute myocardial infarction, can be expected to reduce muscle damage and mortality significantly when thrombolysis has been effective. However much of this still remains to be proven for most of the agents. Since each of the agents are distinctive chemically and pharmacologically, differences are observed in their clinical use. At present, no agent has established superiority over the others as yet, nor does it appear that fibrin binding endows clinical benefits not achievable with the non-fibrin selective agents. Rather each agent and its associated therapeutic regimens has advantages and disadvantages both in terms of risk/benefit and cost/benefit.

This author believes that current research which emphasizes the development of new, more effective agents will prove disappointing in terms of greater clinical benefit. Rather the emphasis should be on developing improved methods for the prevention of the prothrombotic aspects of thrombolytic therapy. Advances in this area could have a major effect in extending the benefits of reperfusion therapy.

Finally thrombolytic therapy will prove of greatest value when treatment is started very early after the onset of the sustained ischemic event. To achieve this on a wide scale will require highly organized and coordinated programs involving patient and physician education and the designing of adequately controlled systems for initiating therapy as soon as possible. This can no longer be left to physicians alone; it is a matter of the public health and deserves the active involvement of all health care agencies.

References

1. Sherry S, Appraisal of various thrombolytic agents in the treatment of acute myocardial infarction. *Am. J. Med. 83* (Supplement 2A), 1987, 31–46.
2. Willerson J T, Winneford M, Buja LM, Thrombolytic therapy for patients with acute myocardial infarction. *Am. J. Med. Sci. 293*, 1987, 187–200.
3. Marder V J, Sherry S, Thrombolytic therapy: current status. *N. Engl. J. Med.* 318, 1988, 1512–1520, 1585–1595.
4. Symposium on Anisoylated Plasminogen Streptokinase Activator Complex (APSAC). Anderson J L, Boissel J P, Chamberlain D A (eds). *Drugs 33* (Supplement 3), 1987, 1–316.
5. Symposium on Modern Thrombolytic Therapy. Braunwald E (ed.). *J. Am. Coll. Cardiol. 10* (Supplement B), 1987, 1B–104B.
6. Symposium on Myocardial Reperfusion 1988: Practical considerations. Topol E J, Califf R M (eds). *J. Am. Coll. Cardiol.* 12 (Supplement A), 1988, 1A–92A.
7. Thrombolysis and the heart. In *Cardiology Clinics*, Sobel B E (ed.), Saunders Co., Philadelphia, 5, 1987, 1–145.
8. *Tissue Plasminogen Activator in Thrombolytic Therapy*, Sobel B E, Collen D, Grossbard E B (eds). Dekker Inc., New York, 1987, 3–241.
9. Kakkar V V, Kennedy W J, Mettinger K L (eds), *Coronary Thrombolytic Therapy*, Current Medical Literature Ltd., London, 1988, 1–158.
10. Sherry S, Schroder R, Kluft C, Six A J, Mettinger K L (eds), *Controversies in Coronary Thrombolysis*, Current Medical Literature Ltd, London, 1989, pp 1–166.
11. Mueller H S, Rao A K, Forman S A, and the TIMI Investigators, Thrombolysis in myocardial infarction (TIMI): Comparative studies of coronary reperfusion and systemic fibrinogenolysis with two forms of recombinant tissue-type plasminogen activator. *J. Am. Coll. Cardiol. 10*, 1987, 479–490.
12. Ferres H, Preclinical pharmacological evaluation of anisoylated plasminogen streptokinase activator complex. *Drugs 33* (Supplement 3), 1987, 33–50.

13. Owen J, Friedman K D, Grossman B A, *et al.*, Quantitation of fragment X formation during thrombolytic therapy with streptokinase and tissue plasminogen activator. *J. Clin. Invest. 79*, 1987, 1642–1647.
14. ISIS–2 (Second International Study of Infarct Survival) Collaborative Group. Randomized trial of intravenous streptokinase, oral aspirin, both or neither among 17,187 cases of suspected acute myocardial infarction: ISIS–2. *Lancet 2*, 1988, 349–360.
15. Yusuf S, Collins R, Peto R, *et al.*, Intravenous and intracoronary fibrinolytic therapy in acute myocardial infarction: overview of results on mortality, reinfarction and side-effects from 33 randomized controlled trials. *Eur. Heart. J. 6*, 1985, 556–585.
16. Stampfer M J, Goldhaber S Z, Yusuf S, *et al.*, Effect of intravenous streptokinase on acute myocardial infarction: pooled results from randomized trials. *N. Engl. J. Med. 307*, 1982, 1180–1182.
17. Kennedy J W, Ritchie J L, Davis K B, Fritz J K, Western Washington Randomized Trial of Intracoronary Streptokinase in Acute Myocardial Infarction, *N. Engl. J. Med. 309*, 1983, 1477–1482.
18. AIMS Trial Study Group. Effect of intravenous APSAC on mortality after acute myocardial infarction: preliminary report of a placebo controlled clinical trial. *Lancet 1*, 1988, 545–549.
19. Kennedy J W, Streptokinase for the treatment of acute myocardial infarction: a brief review of randomized trials. *J. Am. Coll. Cardiol. 10* (Supplement B), 1987, 28B–32B.
20. Dalen J E, Gore J M, Braunwald E, *et al.*, Six- and twelve-month follow-up of the phase I Thrombolysis in Myocardial Infarction (TIMI) Trial. *Am. J. Cardiol. 62*, 1988, 179–185.
21. Sheehan F H, Braunwald E, Canner P, *et al.*, The effect of intravenous thrombolytic therapy on left ventricular function: a report on tissue-type plasminogen activator and streptokinase from the Thrombolysis in Myocardial Infarction (TIMI Phase I) Trial. *Circulation 75*, 1987, 817–829.
22. Chesebro J H, Knatterud G, Roberts R, *et al.*, Thrombolysis in Myocardial Infarction (TIMI) Trial, Phase I: a comparison between intravenous tissue plasminogen activator and intravenous streptokinase. Clinical findings through hospital discharge. *Circulation 76*, 1987, 142–154.
23. Verstraete M, Bleifeld W, Bory M, *et al.*, Randomized trial of intravenous tissue-type plasminogen activator versus intravenous streptokinase in acute myocardial infarction: report from the European Cooperative Study Group for Recombinant Tissue-type Plasminogen Activator. *Lancet 1*, 1985, 842–847.
24. Neuhaus K-L, Tebbe U, Gottwik M, *et al.*, Intravenous recombinant tissue plasminogen activator (rt-PA) and urokinase in acute myocardial infarction: results of the German Activator Urokinase Study (GAUS). *J. Am. Coll Cardiol. 12*, 1988, 581–587.
25. Anderson J L, Rothbard R L, Hackworthy R A, Multicenter reperfusion trial of intravenous anisoylated plasminogen streptokinase activator complex (APSAC) in acute myocardial infarction: controlled comparison with intracoronary streptokinase. *J. Am. Col. Cardiol. 11*, 1988, 1153–1163.
26. Six A J, Dose-effect relationships of streptokinase. In *Controversies in Coronary Thrombolysis*, Sherry S, Schroder R, Kluft C, Six A J, Mettinger K L (eds), Current Medical Literature Ltd., London, 1989, pp 31–40.
27. Sorenson S G, Hackworthy R A, Fitzpatrick P G, *et al.*, Acute coronary occlusion – reliability of angiographic classification and grading. *Drugs 33* (Supplement 3), 1987, 163–168.
28. Jan K-M, Reinhart W, Chien S, *et al.*, Altered rheological properties of blood following administration of tissue plasminogen activator and streptokinase in patients with acute myocardial infarction. *Circulation 72* (Supplement III), 1985, III–417 (Abstract).

29. Arntz R, Heitz J, Schafer H, Schroder R, Hemorheology in acute myocardial infarction: effects of high dose intravenous streptokinase. *Circulation 72* (Supplement III), 1985, III–417 (Abstract).
30. Jan K-M, Chien S, Bigger J T Jr, Observations on blood viscosity changes after acute myocardial infarction. *Circulation 51*, 1975, 1079–1084.
31. European Cooperative Study Group. Streptokinase in acute myocardial infarction. Extended report. In Verstraete M, van de Loo, Jesdinsky H J. Streptokinase in Acute Myocardial Infarction. *Acta. Med Scand. Supplement 648*, 1981, 7–57.
32. White H D, Morris R M, Brown M A, *et al.*, Effect of intravenous streptokinase on left ventricular function and early survival after acute myocardial infarction. *N. Engl. J. Med. 317*, 1987, 850–855.
33. Hall G H, Bolus streptokinase after myocardial infarction. *Lancet 2*, 1987, 96 (Letter to Editor).
34. Sherry S, Dissimilar systemic and local adverse effects of thrombolytic therapy, *Am. J. Cardiol. 61*, 1988, 1344–1346.
35. Golino P, Ashton J H, Glas-Greenwalt P, *et al.*, Mediation of reocclusion by thromboxane A and serotonin after thrombolysis with tissue-type plasminogen activator in a canine preparation of coronary thrombosis. *Circulation 77*, 1988, 678–684.
36. Fitzgerald D J, Catella F, Roy L, FitzGerald G A. Marked platelet activation *in vivo* after intravenous streptokinase in patients with acute myocardial infarction. *Circulation 77*, 1988, 142–150.
37. Rao A K, Pratt C, Berke A, *et al.*, Thrombolysis in Myocardial Infarction (TIMI) Trial – Phase I: hemorrhagic manifestations and changes in plasma fibrinogen and the fibrinolytic system in patients treated with recombinant tissue plasminogen activator and streptokinase. *J. Am Coll. Cardiol. 11*, 1988, 1–11.
38. Fitzgerald D J, FitzGerald G A., Platelet activation by streptokinase: role of plasminogen. *Circulation 76* (Supplement IV), 1987, IV-153 (Abstract).
39. Eisenberg P R, Sherman L A, Jaffe A S, Paradoxic elevation of fibrinopeptide A after streptokinase: evidence for continued thrombosis despite intense fibrinolysis. *J. Am. Coll. Cardiol. 10*, 1987, 527–530.
40. Lee C D, Mann K G, The activation of human coagulation factor V by plasmin. *Blood 70* (Supplement 1), 1987, 389a (Abstract).
41. Atkinson J L D, Sundt T M, Kazmier F J, *et al.*, Heparin-induced thrombocytopenia and thrombosis in ischemic stroke. *Mayo Clin Proc. 63*, 1988, 353–361.
42. Sobel M, Adelman B, Platelet activation enhances heparin binding. *Blood 70* (Supplement 1), 1987, 361a (Abstract).
43. Teitel J M, Rosenberg R D, Protection of Factor Xa from neutralization by the heparin-antithrombin complex. *J. Clin. Invest. 71*, 1983, 1383–1391.
44. Gold H K, Leinbach R C, Garabedian H D, *et al.*, Acute coronary reocclusion after thrombolysis with recombinant tissue-type plasminogen activator: prevention by a maintenance infusion. *Circulation 73*, 1986, 347–352.
45. Johns J A, Gold H K, Leinbach R C, et al., Prevention of coronary artery reocclusion and reduction in late coronary artery stenosis after thrombolytic therapy in patients with acute myocardial infarction: A randomized study of maintenance infusion of recombinant human tissue-type plasminogen activator. *Circulation 78*, 1988, 546–556.
46. TIMI Operations Committee. Announcement of protocol change in thrombolysis in myocardial infarction trial. *J. Am. Coll. Cardiol.* 9, 1987, 467 (Letter to Editor).
47. Van de Werf F, for the Investigators of the European Cooperative Study Group for Recombinant Tissue-type Plasminogen Activator. Lessons from the European Cooperative

Recombinant Tissue-type Plasminogen Activator (rt-PA) Versus Placebo Trial. *J. Am. Coll. Cardiol. 12* (Supplement A), 1988, 14A–19A.
48. Sasahara A A, Hyers T M, Cole C M, *et al.*, The Urokinase Pulmonary Embolism Trial, a national cooperative study. *Circulation 47* (Supplement II), 1974, II-1 – II-108.
49. Marder V J, Relevance of changes in blood fibrinolytic and coagulation parameters during thrombolytic therapy. *Am. J. Med. 83* (Supplement 2a), 1987, 15–19.
50. Urokinase-Streptokinase Embolism Trial: phase 2 results: a cooperative study. *J.A M.A. 229*, 1974, 1606–1613.
51. Francis C W, Markham R E Jr, Barlow G H, *et al.*, Thrombin activity of fibrin thrombi and soluble plasmic derivatives. *J. Lab. Clin. Med. 102*, 1983, 220–230.
52. Ohlstein E H, Storer B, Fujita T, Shebuski R J. Tissue-type plasminogen activator and streptokinase induced platelet hyperaggregatability in the rabbit. *Thromb. Res. 46*, 1987, 574–586.
53. Gold H K, Coller B S, Yasuda T, *et al.*, Rapid and sustained coronary artery recanalization with combined bolus injection of recombinant tissue-type plasminogen activator and monoclonal antiplatelet GP IIb/IIIa antibody in a canine preparation. *Circulation 77*, 1988, 670–677.
54. White H D, Rivers J T, Maslowski A H, *et al.*, Effect of intravenous streptokinase as compared to that of tissue plasminogen activator on left ventricular function after first myocardial infarction. *N. Engl. J. Med. 320*, 1989, 817–821.
55. Magnani B. for the PAIMS Investigators. Plasminogen activator Italian Multicenter Study (PAIMS): Comparison of intravenous recombinant single-chain human tissue-type plasminogen activator (rt-PA) with intravenous streptokinase in acute myocardial infarction. *J. Am. Coll. Cardiol. 13*, 1989, 19–26.
56. Durand P, Asseman P, Pruvost P, *et al.*, Effectiveness of intravenous streptokinase on infarct size and left ventricular function in acute myocardial infarction. Prospective and randomized study. *Clin. Cardiol. 10*, 1987, 383–393.
57. Kennedy J W, Martin G V, Davis K B, *et al.*, The Western Washington Intravenous Streptokinase in Acute Myocardial Infarction Randomized Trial. *Circulation 77*, 1988, 345–352.
58. The I.S.A.M. Study Group. A prospective trial of intravenous streptokinase in acute myocardial infarction (I.S.A.M.). Mortality, morbidity, and infarct size at 21 days. *N. Engl. J. Med. 314*, 1986, 1465–1471.
59. Schreiber T L, Miller D H, Silvasi D A, *et al.*, Randomized double-blind trial of intravenous streptokinase for acute myocardial infarction. *Am. J. Cardiol. 58*, 1986, 47–52.
60. Bassand J P, Faivre R, Becque O, *et al.*, Intravenous streptokinase versus heparin in recent acute myocardial infarction. Multicentre randomized trial in the Franche Comté Area. *Haemostasis* 16 (Supplement 3), 1986, 130–139.
61. Guerci A D, Gerstenblith G, Brinker J A, *et al.*, A randomized trial of intravenous tissue plasminogen activator for acute myocardial infarction with subsequent randomization to elective angioplasty. *N. Engl. J. Med. 317*, 1987, 1613–1618.
62. National Heart Foundation of Australia Coronary Thrombolysis Group. Coronary thrombolysis and myocardial salvage by tissue plasminogen activator given up to 4 hours after onset of myocardial infarction. *Lancet 1*, 1988, 203–207.
63. O'Rourke M, Baron D, Keogh A, *et al.*, Limitation of myocardial infarction by early infusion of recombinant tissue-type plasminogen activator. *Circulation 77*, 1988, 1311–1315.
64. Bassand J-P, Machecourt J, Cassagnes J, *et al.*, Multicenter trial of intravenous anisoylated plasminogen streptokinase activator complex (APSAC) in acute myocardial infarction:

Effects on infarct size and left ventricular function. *J. Am. Coll. Cardiol. 13*, 1989, 988–997.

65. Gruppo Italiano per lo Studio della Streptochinasi Nell'Infarto Miocardico (GISSI). Effectiveness of intravenous thrombolytic treatment in acute myocardial infarction. *Lancet 1*, 1986, 397–402.
66. Gruppo Italiano per lo Studio della Streptochinasi nell'Infarto Miocardico (GISSI). Long-term effects of intravenous thrombolysis in acute myocardial infarction: final report of the GISSI study. *Lancet 2*, 1987, 871–874.
67. Wilcox R G, von der Lippe G, Olsson C G, *et al.*, Trial of tissue plasminogen activator for mortality reduction in acute myocardial infarction. Anglo-Scandinavian Study of Early Thrombolysis (ASSET). *Lancet 2*, 1988, 525–530.
68. Antiplatelet Trialists' Collaboration. Secondary prevention of vascular disease by prolonged antiplatelet treatment. *Brit. Med. J. 296*, 1988, 320–331.
69. Sherry S, Unresolved clinical pharmacologic questions in thrombolytic therapy for acute myocardial infarction. *J. Am. Coll. Cardiol. 12*, 1988, 519–525.

Chapter 2

THE ANGLO-SCANDINAVIAN STUDY OF EARLY THROMBOLYSIS (ASSET): A TRIAL OF TISSUE PLASMINOGEN ACTIVATOR FOR MORTALITY REDUCTION IN PATIENTS WITH SUSPECTED ACUTE MYOCARDIAL INFARCTION

J. R. Hampton and R. G. Wilcox

University Hospital, Nottingham, UK

Summary

In the Anglo-Scandinavian Study of Early Thrombolysis (ASSET) 13,318 patients admitted to 52 coronary care units with suspected acute myocardial infarction were considered for inclusion in a double-blind study comparing recombinant tissue-type plasminogen activator (rt-PA) 100 mg plus heparin with placebo plus heparin. 8307 (62%) were excluded, mainly because their symptoms had begun more than 5 h previously, but all excluded patients were followed up at least until hospital discharge. 2516 patients were randomly allocated to rt-PA and 2495 to placebo. At one month the overall case fatality rates were 7.2% and 9.8% respectively, a relative reduction of 26% (95% confidence interval 11 to 39%). 6.3% of patients given rt-PA had a bleeding complication (1.4% major) compared with 0.8% given placebo (0.4% major).

The results of ASSET are compared with those of the other major thrombolytic trials in which fatality rate was the main endpoint.

Introduction

Tissue plasminogen activator, produced by recombinant technology, (rt-PA) has theoretical advantages over streptokinase and anisoylated streptokinase-plasminogen activator complex (anistreplase, formerly known as APSAC): rt-PA is not antigenic and does not cause rashes or anaphylactic reactions, and being more fibrin-specific it has less effect on circulating fibrinogen and other clotting factors.[1,2] rt-PA should therefore be safer than products related to streptokinase. Moreover, angiographic studies have shown that it leads to higher rates of early patency in coronary arteries after myocardial infarction than does streptokinase.[2,3,4] rt-PA might therefore be the most effective of the thrombolytic agents for the reduction of fatality in patients with myocardial infarction.

The Anglo-Scandinavian Study of Early Thrombolysis (ASSET) was designed and commenced before the results of the main studies of streptokinase and anistreplase (ISIS-2 and AIMS)[5,6] were available, and the value of thrombolysis in acute myocardial infarction was at that time still not established. ASSET was therefore designed as a placebo-controlled trial, not as a direct comparison of rt-PA with any other thrombolytic agents.

This paper describes the main results of ASSET, and in an attempt to compare the efficacy of rt-PA with the other thrombolytic agents compares the design and results of ASSET with the design and results of the other major thrombolytic trials. A full description of the results of ASSET has been published elsewhere.[7]

The design of ASSET

Patients and methods

Inclusion and exclusion criteria

All patients admitted to the coronary care unit (CCUs) of the participating centres with suspected myocardial infarction were registered and considered for inclusion.

Patients of either sex could be included in the study if they were aged 18 to 75 years and if acute myocardial infarction was suspected clinically. No electrocardiographic (ECG) criteria were required. Patients were considered for inclusion only if treatment with rt-PA (or placebo) could begin within 5 h of the onset of major symptoms. Patients were excluded if there was a history suggesting any risk of bleeding.

Trial medication and randomization

Randomization was achieved within each centre by taking the next pack of trial medication from a numbered sequence, in which active and placebo therapies were in random order in blocks of 20. An included patient was treated with the next pack in the sequence. rt-PA was given as a bolus dose of 10 mg followed by an infusion of 50 mg in 1 h and then 20 mg in each of the next 2 h. The same procedure was followed with the placebo material. All patients were given an initial bolus dose of intravenous heparin 5000 units, and, after administration of rt-PA or placebo, a heparin infusion of 1000 units/h was administered for 21 h.

All centres followed a common therapeutic policy for uncomplicated cases. During the hospital stay intravenous beta-blockers, prophylactic antiarrhythmic agents, and anticoagulants other than specified by the trial protocol were not used. After discharge a prophylactic beta-blocker was permitted, but anticoagulants, aspirin and other anti-platelet drugs were not given. Exercise testing and coronary angiography were done only in patients with persisting symptoms.

Follow-up

All patients have been followed for 6 months. This account is concerned only with results to the end of the first month.

In the UK and some Scandinavian centres all excluded patients were followed up to 1 month from admission; in the remainder follow-up was limited to the time of hospital discharge.

Trial administration

Fifty-two centres in the UK, Norway, Sweden, and Denmark took part. The trial was coordinated from the department of medicine, Nottingham University. In the four countries a national coordinator organized the groups of investigators, helped by an employee of Boehringer Ingelheim. Major decisions were taken by a steering committee (chairman, international coordinator, and national coordinators); company personnel usually attended as observers. Data were handled by the Department of Mathematics, Nottingham University, independently of the trial Steering Committee and the sponsoring company. The trial results were monitored by an independent ethical committee who would have advised premature termination of the study if predetermined differences between the treatment groups had been observed. These 'stopping rules' were not needed.

Statistical methods

The only end-point was death. It was assumed that the 1-month overall fatality rate in the placebo group would be 12% and that the 6-month overall fatality rate in the placebo group would be 15%. A trial in 5000 patients would thus have greater than 90% power to detect a relative difference of 20% between the rt-PA and placebo groups at 6 months and would be large enough to examine mortality both at 6 months and at 1 month.

Results

Recruitment

Recruitment began in England and Norway in November 1986, in Sweden in April 1987, and in Denmark in autumn, 1987. Seventeen English, eleven Norwegian, fifteen Swedish, and nine Danish hospitals took part. By the time recruitment was stopped on 29 February 1988, 13,318 consecutive patients with suspected acute myocardial infarction had been considered for the study. 8307 (62%) were excluded (Table 1). Of the 8148 fully documented excluded patients, 4944 (61%) had an in-hospital diagnosis of myocardial infarction, 1890 (23%) ischaemic heart disease without myocardial infarction, 798 (10%) chest pain for which no cause could be found, and 516 (6%) other diagnoses. Overall mortality was 13.1%. In the patients with myocardial infarction mortality was 17.1%, in those with ischaemic heart disease without myocardial infarction 2.4%, in those with chest pain for which no cause could be found 1%, and in those with other diagnoses 6.5%.

Included patients

Of 13,318 consecutive patients, 5011 (37.6%) were randomized to placebo plus heparin (2495) or rt-PA plus heparin (2516). By 1 June 1988, the 1 month outcome was known for 5009 patients (one patient from each group was lost from local follow-up after hospital discharge). The following results are derived from 5005 fully documented patients (rt-PA 2512, placebo 2493), except for 1 month mortality which considers 5009 randomized patients.

The two treatment groups were well matched and the interval between onset of major symptoms and start of treatment was similar in the two groups (1 h or less 2%, 1–2 h 11%, 2–3 h 26%, 3–4 h 29%, 4–5 h 27%, over 5 h 4%). After randomization 265 (10.5%) patients in the rt-PA group and 152 (6.1%) in the placebo group had their trial infusion or heparin prematurely terminated. Although there was a significant excess of bleeding in the rt-PA group this rarely required specific action such as replacement transfusion.

Outcome at 1 month

The in-hospital diagnostic categorization was similar in the two groups with a slight shift towards fewer definite infarcts in the rt-PA group (Table 2). There was very little difference in either cardiovascular complications or cardiovascular treatment, apart from cardiogenic shock (p 0.05). There was no difference in the emergence of ventricular arrhythmias necessitating drug treatment or defibrillation (Table 3).

Table 1 *Reasons for exclusion from the study, expressed as a percentage of the 8148 excluded patients for whom data is available*

Duration of symptoms greater than 5 hours	73.5%
Age greater than 75 years	8.3%
Refused	4.3%
Pregnancy	0.3%
High systolic blood pressure	2.2%
Recent stroke, trauma or surgery	3.6%
Proliferative retinopathy	1.5%
Recent haemorrhage, known peptic ulceration or bleeding diathesis	6.1%
Emergency cardiac massage	4.1%
Sensitivity to gentamycin	0.1%
Already receiving warfarin	4.2%
Other serious concomitant disease	5.4%
Unable to attend for local follow-up	3.6%

Table 2 *Hospital discharge diagnostic categorization (%)*

	rt-PA No.	*(2512)* %	*Placebo* No.	*(2493)* %
Myocardial infarction	1811	(72.1)	1783	(71.5)
IHD	429	(17.0)	426	(17.0)
Chest pain of unknown cause	198	(7.8)	202	(8.1)
Other diagnosis	73	(2.9)	81	(3.2)
Missing data	1		1	

Table 3 *In-hospital complications other than strokes (%)*

	rt-PA		*Placebo*	
	No.	*%*	*No.*	*%*
Recurrent MI	99	3.9	114	4.5
Ventricular fibrillation	94	3.7	116	4.6
Asystole	100	3.9	122	4.8
Pulmonary embolism	11	0.4	14	0.5
Other embolism	12	0.4	19	0.7
Cardiogenic shock	96	3.8	129	5.1 $p<0.05$
Heart failure	446	17.7	461	18.4

Total patient population 13,318

Entered 5,011 — 8,307 Excluded (see text)

rt-PA 2,516 — Placebo 2,495

	rt-PA continued	rt-PA withdrawn	Placebo continued	Placebo withdrawn
	2,287	229	2,384	111
Missing	1			1
No. of deaths	135	47	204	41
% Dead	5.9	20.5	8.5	37.2
Total dead	182/2,515		245/2494	
% Dead	7.2		9.8	

Figure 1 *Fatality rates after one month*

By 1 month 7.2% of patients given rt-PA and 9.8% of those given placebo had died (relative reduction 26%; 95% confidence interval (CI) 11 to 39%; p = 0.0011). Patients withdrawn before the completion of the trial infusion had a case fatality rate higher than did those who continued, irrespective of trial allocation (Fig. 1).

At 1 month 282 rt-PA patients and 257 placebo patients who had been discharged had been readmitted with a similar pattern of diagnoses. There was also a comparable proportion of 1 month survivors with either angina (rt-PA 30%, placebo 29%) or heart failure (rt-PA 18%, placebo 20%). There was no excess of patients in the rt-PA group with delayed reinfarction.

Adverse events

Adverse events were separately recorded, but they did not necessarily lead to premature termination of either the trial infusion or the subsequent infusion of heparin. The greatest difference between the two groups was the significant excess in the rt-PA group of both major bleeds and minor bleeds (Table 4). Strokes were categorized by clinical, computerized tomographic (CT) scan, or post-mortem diagnosis. By 1 month there had been 28 patients with strokes in the rt-PA group (1.1%) of whom 11 died, giving a risk of death from stroke of 0.4%. In the placebo group there were 25 strokes and six deaths, giving a stroke incidence of 1.0% and a risk of death from stroke of 0.2%. More of the strokes in the rt-PA group occurred during the first 24 hours compared with the placebo group, half of them being classified as haemorrhagic (Table 5).

There were eight dissecting aortic aneurysms in the rt-PA group. Five were recognized during the first 24 hours and were fatal within 48 h; two occurred later in the hospital stay and the patients survived to 1 month; and another patient survived a dissection between hospital discharge and 1 month. There were five aortic aneurysms in the placebo group and all were diagnosed in hospital – two during the infusion period (one died) and three later on (one died).

Subset analysis

The intention-to-treat analysis of the included patients is shown in the figure. Most of the deaths were in patients with an in-hospital diagnosis of AMI (93% of rt-PA deaths, 96% of placebo deaths). The 1 month fatality rate in those with a diagnosis of infarction was 9% in the rt-PA

Table 4 *Number of patients with adverse events*

	rt-PA	*Placebo*
Cardiac	192	185
Major bleeds	35	12
Minor bleeds	158	8
Other adverse events	27	30

Table 5 *Strokes according to time and treatment*

	rt-PA		*Placebo*	
	during infusion	*post infusion*	*during infusion*	*post infusion*
Haemorrhagic (dead)	6 (5)	1	–	2 (2)
Embolic	3 (1)	8 (2)	2 (1)	15 (2)
Unclassified	3 (2)	7 (1)		6 (1)
Total	12 (8)	16 (3)	2 (1)	23 (5)

group and 13% in the placebo group (relative reduction 28%, 95% CI 14–41%). (Table 6). Patients admitted with an unequivocally normal ECG had a 1 month fatality rate of 1.6% if given rt-PA and of 3.0% if given placebo; among those who had an abnormal ECG on admission the fatality rate was 8.5% in the rt-PA group and 11.2% in those given placebo (relative reduction 24.5%, 95% CI 9–37%).

The patients were not separately stratified according to the time from onset of symptoms to start of trial treatment and only 2% were entered within an hour. There was no consistent effect of rt-PA according to delay before treatment, and the overall outcome at 1 month was similar in those treated within 3 h of the onset of symptoms or between 3 and 5 h (Table 7). Patients were not stratified either by age or sex. There was little difference between the sexes in terms of improvement with rt-PA, but analysis by age suggested an increasing benefit from rt-PA treatment with increasing age (Table 7).

Table 6 *Subset analysis – outcome at one month by initial ECG*

	rt-PA		*Placebo*	
ECG	*No.*	*Deaths*	*No.*	*Deaths*
Normal	443	7 (1.6%)	431	13 (3.0%)
Abnormal	2607	175 (8.5%)	2026	231 (11.2%)
Missing	2	–	–	–

Comparison of ASSET and the other main thrombolytic trials

The results of ASSET show clearly that rt-PA reduces fatality in patients with suspected myocardial infarction. ASSET was designed as a placebo-controlled trial, and no direct comparison of the different thrombolytic agents using mortality as an endpoint has yet been published. Comparing the thrombolytic trials in an attempt to determine which agent leads to the greatest reduction in fatality is fraught with difficulty, and may well be misleading but neverthless it is important for immediate clinical practice to know whether any of the agents appears superior. We need to compare the trials not only in terms of outcome, but also in terms of their design and the patients included if we are to come to any conclusions as to whether any sort of comparison is valid.

Five large trials with mortality as an endpoint have now been published, three using SK, one using APSAC and one rt-PA. These trials are usually referred to by their acronyms: ISAM[8] (Intravenous SK in acute myocardial infarction), GISSI[9,10] (Gruppo Italiano per lo Studio della Streptochinasi nell'Infarto miocardico), ISIS-2[5] (Second International Study of Infarct Survival), AIMS[6] (the APSAC Infarction Mortality Study) and ASSET.[7]

Table 8 shows the total number of patients in each trial. The AIMS study was smallest because recruitment was terminated when the ethical committee supervising the study found that the difference in outcome between the treated and placebo groups had reached the limit defined as acceptable in the protocol (the 'stopping rule').

The ISAM, GISSI, and ASSET studies were all of conventional design and were pursued to their intended recruitment total. GISSI was unlike the others in being an open study, but with centralized randomization to prevent bias and perhaps because of this, full data on the control group have not been provided. The ISAM and ASSET studies were simple in concept, but the patient records were reasonably detailed. ISIS-2, and to a lesser extent GISSI aimed to collect minimal data.

ISIS-2 was unique in attempting to answer two questions at once by means of a factorial design. As well as studying the effect of SK the trial aimed to determine whether aspirin has a protective effect in patients with myocardial infarction. Patients were therefore randomized to one of four groups – SK only, aspirin only, SK plus aspirin, or placebo. The groups were then combined so that those patients given SK were compared with those that were not, and those

Table 7 *Subset analysis – outcome at one month by time to treatment, sex and age*

	rt-PA			*Placebo*		
	No.	*Dead*	*% Dead*	*No.*	*Dead*	*% Dead*
Time 0–3 hr.	992	81	8.1	979	107	10.9
> 3 hr.	1504	99	6.5	1488	129	8.6
missing	16	2		26	8	
Men	1935	132	6.8	1928	182	9.4
Women	576	50	8.6	565	62	10.9
Age ≤ 55	748	29	3.8	745	33	4.4
−65	963	63	6.5	896	71	7.9
−75	827	90	10.8	852	140	16.4

given aspirin were compared with those given aspirin placebo, in each case the use of aspirin or SK respectively being ignored. The effect of aspirin was clearly demonstrated, but because of the way the data have been presented it is difficult to disentangle the effects of SK and aspirin.

Table 9 shows some of the other differences in the design of these major trials. In ISIS-2 and ASSET, patients could be included if a myocardial infarction was suspected but the ECG was normal: the aim was to include patients as soon as possible after the onset of symptoms, at a time when the ECG might still be normal.

In some ways the differences between the trials are useful because they illuminate different aspects of thrombolytic therapy. In other ways, however, the differences make it difficult to compare the trial results. If we are to compare the efficacy of the different thrombolytic agents we need to be confident that similar patients were included in each trial. Differences in 'inclusion criteria' shown in Table 9 make some variation between the trials inevitable, but the 'exclusion criteria' were essentially the same in all studies for it was commonly felt that patients with recent trauma, surgery, a stroke, or who had any possible bleeding tendency, should not be given thrombolytic treatment.

The best indication of whether or not the trial patients were similar is given by the fatality rate in the different placebo groups. Table 10 shows that there was remarkable similarity in the placebo group fatality rates in the different trials with those in GISSI, AIMS, and ISIS-2 being respectively 13.0, 12.2 and 13.0%. In ISAM the fatality rate was low at 7.1%. In ASSET 9.8% of the placebo group died but this trial was unusual in including a relatively high proportion (17%) of patients with a normal ECG and if these are excluded (thus making the placebo group

Table 8 *The major thrombolysis trials with mortality as the main endpoint*

Trial	*Thrombolytic agent and dose*	*Total number of patients included*
ISAM	SK 1.5 MU	1,741
GISSI	SK 1.5 MU	11,806
ISIS-2	SK 1.5 MU	17,187
AIMS	Anistreplase (APSAC) 30 u	1,004
ASSET	rt-PA 100 mg	5,011

Table 9 *Differences in the protocols of the thrombolysis trials*

	Age limit (years)	*Maximum delay (hours)*	*ECG abnormalities required*	*Patient register*
ISAM	75	6	yes	yes
GISSI	any age	12	yes	yes
ISIS-2	any age	24	no	no
AIMS	70	6	yes	no
ASSET	75	5	no	yes

Table 10 *Comparison of patients included in placebo groups of thrombolysis trials*

	Age (years)	*Delay <3 hours (%)*	*Placebo group fatality rate (%)*
ISAM	> 70 18%	52	3 weeks 7.1%
GISSI	> 65 36%	53	3 weeks 13.0%
ISIS-2	> 70 20%	29*	5 weeks 13.0%
AIMS	> 60 40%	< 4 hours 60%	4 weeks 12.2%
ASSET	> 65 34%	39	4 weeks 9.8%**

* In ISIS-2, 41% of those admitted within six hours had symptoms of less than 3 hours' duration.
** In ASSET the fatality rate for those with abnormal ECGs on admission was 11.8%.

more similar to those in the other trials) the fatality rate increases to 11.2%. It therefore seems probable that similar patients were included in all the studies.

Table 11 shows the differences in fatality between the groups of patients given active or placebo treatment. The figures of ISIS-2 refer to those given SK alone and those given only placebo therapy; patients given aspirin are not included.

In each trial active treatment reduced the numbers of deaths and the relative reduction compared with placebo ranged from 11% (ISAM) to 47% (AIMS). The ISAM result was the only one that was not statistically significant.

Table 11 also shows the 95% confidence intervals for the point estimates of relative risk reduction. The smaller the trial the wider are the confidence intervals, so the 'true' results of ISAM and AIMS could lie within a wide range. The confidence intervals all overlap, and the effect of SK in ISAM might actually have been as good as that of anistreplase (APSAC) in AIMS. It is important to realize, however, that an overlap of the confidence intervals around the observed results of different trials does not mean that the treatments were identical; the only conclusion that can be drawn from overlapping confidence intervals is that the trials were not large enough, or that the differences between their results were too small for the studies to have the power to detect any difference.

There is thus no evidence in these trials to suggest that one treatment is different from another. The marked difference in the point estimates of the results of ISAM and ISIS-2 (11% and 22% relative reduction respectively) shows what can occur in different trials when identical treatment regimens are used in apparently similar patients, and this must lead to extreme caution in suggesting that the 47% relative reduction of risk seen in AIMS represents any real difference between APSAC and SK.

Conclusions

ASSET demonstrated that rt-PA is a safe and effective thrombolytic agent in patients with suspected myocardial infarction. The main advantage of ASSET in comparison with the other

Table 11 *Effect of thrombolytic treatment on fatality*

	Placebo		*Active*		*Relative reduction*	*95% CI*
	No.	*%*	*No.*	*%*	*(%)*	*(%)*
ISAM	882	7.1	859	6.3	11.3	−22 to + 44
GISSI	5852	13.0	5860	10.7	18	10–28
ISIS 2 (SK vs. placebo)	4300	13.0	4300	10.3	22	16–28
AIMS	502	12.2	502	6.4	47	21–65
ASSET	2495	9.8	2516	7.2	26	11–39

major thrombolytic trials was in the detailed register of patients who were excluded from the study, but whose outcome was known, so that the general applicability of the ASSET results can easily be judged. The reduction in fatality associated with rt-PA therapy was comparable to that seen with other thrombolytic agents. Despite some differences in trial design the major thrombolytic studies can be seen as broadly comparable, and probably included very similar patients. Since the confidence intervals of the results of all the major trials overlap, it is not possible to be certain whether there are any differences in efficacy between the different thrombolytic agents, and this answer can only come from very large clinical trials in which the agents are directly compared.

References

1. van de Werf F, Collen D, Coronary thrombolysis with tissue-type plasminogen activator: an overview. *Eur. Heart. J. 6*, 1985, 902–904.
2. Verstraete M, Bernard R, Bory M, *et al.*, Randomised trial of intravenous recombinant tissue-type plasminogen activator versus intravenous streptokinase in acute myocardial infarction. *Lancet 1*, 1985, 842–847
3. Verstraete M, Bleifeld W, Brower R W, *et al.*, Double-blind randomised trial of intravenous tissue-type plasminogen activator versus placebo in acute myocardial infarction. *Lancet 2*, 1985, 965–969.
4. The TIMI Study Group. The Thrombolysis in myocardial infarction (TIMI) Trial phase I findings. *N. Engl. J. Med. 312*, 1985, 932–936.
5. ISIS-2 (Second International Study of Infarct Survival). Collaborative Group. Randomised trial of intravenous streptokinase, oral aspirin, both, or neither among 17,187 cases of suspected acute myocardial infarction: ISIS-2. *Lancet 2*, 1988, 349–360.
6. AIMS Trial Study Group. Effect of intravenous APSAC on mortality after acute myocardial infarction: preliminary report of a placebo-controlled clinical trial. *Lancet 1*, 1988, 545–549.
7. Wilcox R G, Olsson C G, Skene A M, von der Lippe G, Jensen G, Hampton J R. (For the ASSET Study Group). Trial of tissue plasminogen activator for mortality reduction in acute myocardial infarction. The Anglo-Scandinavian Study of Early Thrombolysis (ASSET). *Lancet 2*, 1988, 525–530.
8. The ISAM Study Group. A prospective trial of intravenous streptokinase in acute myocar-

dial infarction. (ISAM): mortality, morbidity, and infarct size at 21 days. *N. Engl. J. Med. 314*, 1986, 1465–1471.

9. Gruppo Italiano per lo Studio della Streptochinasi nell'Infarto Miocardico (GISSI). Effectiveness of intravenous thrombolytic treatment in acute myocardial infarction. *Lancet 2*, 1986, 397–402.
10. Gruppo Italiano per lo Studio della Streptochinasi nell'Infarto Miocardico (GISSI). Long-term effects of intravenous thrombolysis in acute myocardial infarction Final report of the GISSI Study. *Lancet 2*, 1987, 871–874.

Chapter 3

ANISTREPLASE (APSAC): A REVIEW OF CLINICAL DATA

R. J. Cregeen and Vanda M. McCartney

Beecham Pharmaceuticals, Reigate, UK

Anistreplase (Eminase*), the anisoylated derivative of the human lys-plasminogen streptokinase activator complex – often abbreviated to APSAC, is a novel thrombolytic agent. Clinical studies have clearly demonstrated the efficacy and safety of APSAC in the treatment of acute myocardial infarction (AMI).

Rationale for the development of Anistreplase (APSAC)

The objective in using plasminogen activators to treat patients with acute myocardial infarction (AMI) is to achieve rapid and complete lysis of the occlusive coronary thrombus. Streptokinase forms a powerful plasminogen activator complex when it combines with circulating glu-plasminogen. Consideration was given as to how the properties of this highly active complex could be improved upon or placed under greater control for therapeutic gain.

It was conceived that temporary chemical protection of a key site within the catalytic centre would produce an inert pro-enzyme whose activation *in vivo* and pharmacokinetic disposition

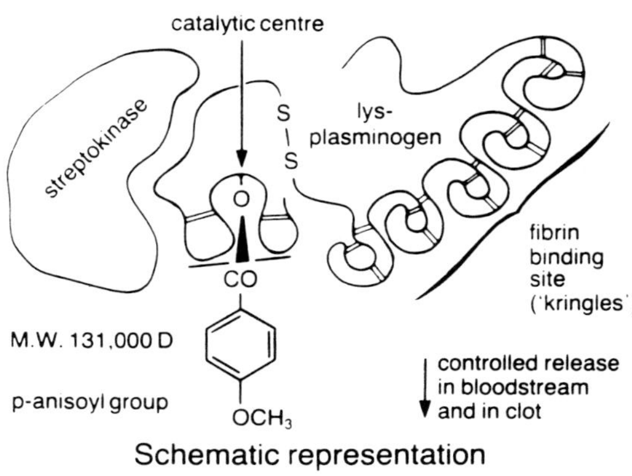

Figure 1 *Anisoylated lys-plasminogen streptokinase activator complex*

*Eminase is a registered trade mark.

would be controlled by the choice of chemical substituent.[1] Synthetic techniques were exploited whereby chemical protection of the catalytic centre would not interfere with other important aspects of the enzyme such as its ability to bind to fibrin via the kringle domain in the molecule. (Fig. 1).

There was a choice whether to use native glu-plasminogen which combines with streptokinase, or a different form, lys-plasminogen, which has a higher affinity for fibrin.

An anisoyl group was chosen to protect, temporarily, the catalytic centre of the enzyme complex and the lys-plasminogen component was selected to improve upon fibrin affinity.

Pharmacological properties

The conversion of anistreplase to its active form occurs by deacylation (removal of anisoyl group) starting immediately after administration and proceeding in a sustained and controlled manner until completion (*in vitro* half life approx 1.75 h).[2]

Acylation of the catalytic centre extends the duration of the fibrinolytic activity of the activator complex over that of the unacylated form. The half-life of fibrinolytic activity in patients with AMI is about 1½ to 2 h for anistreplase and 15–20 minutes for streptokinase.[3,4] Fibrinolytic activity can be detected in the bloodstream for between 6 and 9 hours following anistreplase administration. The prolonged circulation of anistreplase in the bloodstream allows continuous uptake by a thrombus and maintains the thrombolytic action of the drug. The pharmacokinetic profile of anistreplase is consistent with reducing the tendency for early re-thrombosis.

Other thrombolytics have significantly shorter plasma half-lives than anistreplase, i.e the half-lives of streptokinase and urokinase are in the order of 15–20 min, while those of recombinant tissue-type plasminogen activator (t-PA) and single chain urokinase-type plasminogen activator (scu-PA, pro-urokinase) are even shorter, about 5 minutes.[5–8] Hence these agents must be administered by intravenous infusions of various complexities over a minimum of 1 hour to compensate for their pharmacokinetics and to avoid unacceptable reocclusion rates.

In contrast the pharmacokinetic properties of anistreplase allow it to be administered as a single intravenous injection over 2–5 min, yielding major advantages in ease of administration. There is compelling evidence that the benefits of thrombolytic agents are increased by early administration. The ease of administration of anistreplase may allow it to be used earlier than other agents, potentially before admission to hospital.

Thus anistreplase offers advantages in the treatment of acute myocardial infarction with respect to ease of administration and duration of action.

Clinical efficacy

The benefit of anistreplase therapy has been assessed and established in patients presenting with symptoms and signs of AMI, in terms of rates of reperfusion, patency and reocclusion, limitation of infarct size, preservation of left ventricular function, and survival.

In these clinical studies, anistreplase was administered as a standard dose of 30 Units (U) by intravenous injection over 2–5 minutes. This dose was selected on the basis of early dose-ranging work.[9,10]

Selection criteria for patients recruited into the phase III clinical programme were: onset of major symptoms suggestive of AMI within the preceding 4 or 6 hours (depending on specific protocol); chest pain of at least 30 minutes' duration; ECG evidence of AMI (ST segment elevation greater than 0.1 mV in standard leads or 0.2 mV in chest leads); chest pain not reversed by nitrates (in majority of studies); age 70 years or under; no contra-indications to thrombolytic therapy. Anticoagulation therapy was given, beginning 3–6 hours after the administration of trial therapy in the majority of studies. Aspirin was not given routinely in any of these studies.

Reperfusion

The immediate objective of thrombolytic therapy in acute myocardial infarction is to lyse thrombi and restore flow in the infarct related artery thereby restoring the blood supply of the ischaemic tissue. Reperfusion can be directly assessed by coronary angiography performed prior to thrombolytic therapy to demonstrate the presence of an occlusive thrombus in the infarct related coronary artery (IRCA) and after therapy to establish that reperfusion of the artery has occurred. The time to reperfusion can be determined by means of serial angiograms performed at intervals after therapy.

The term 'reperfusion study' refers only those studies that included both pre-treatment and post-treatment coronary angiography. Only patients with demonstrable occlusion at pre-treatment coronary angiography were included in such studies. In these studies, the angiograms were read by independent assessors who were blinded with respect to treatment given.

In randomized comparative studies, reperfusion rates of between 50 and 68% have been reported in patients receiving anistreplase within 6 hours of symptom onset.

In one double-blind, placebo-controlled study, anistreplase given over 2 to 5 minutes was compared with placebo in 40 patients with MI.[11] Twenty-nine patients (16 allocated anistreplase, 13 placebo) had an occluded infarct-related coronary artery (IRCA) at pre-treatment coronary angiography. The mean time to treatment in this group was 3.3 ± 1.3 hours after the onset of symptoms. Reperfusion occurred within 90 minutes in 9/16 (56%) patients who received anistreplase and 1/13 (8%) who were given placebo ($p < 0.05$).

Two further reperfusion studies conducted in North America and the Netherlands, compared anistreplase with intracoronary (i.c.) streptokinase (160,000 to 250,000 IU) long regarded as a 'gold standard' for thrombolytic therapy.[12,13]

In the American Study,[12] 240 qualifying patients with proven coronary occlusion (TIMI grade 0 or 1) were randomized to treatment (either 30 U anistreplase intravenously over 2–4 minutes, or 160,000 IU streptokinase, by intracoronary infusion over 60 minutes) within 6 hours of symptom onset. Reperfusion was evaluated angiographically over 90 minutes and success was defined as advancement from grade 0 or 1 occlusion to grade 2 or 3 flow. Reperfusion at any time within 90 minutes was observed in 55% (67/122) of anistreplase-treated patients and 64% (73/114) of intracoronary streptokinase-treated patients.

In those patients treated within 4 hours, there were similar reperfusion rates in the anistreplase and the intracoronary streptokinase group (59% and 60% respectively). In those patients treated 4 to 6 hours after the onset of symptoms, there were lower reperfusion rates in the anistreplase than the intracoronary streptokinase-treated group (33% versus 61%). Although no time dependency was noted for intracoronary streptokinase, the same time dependency in terms of reperfusion has been noted for intravenous streptokinase.[14,15]

It is also important to note that, in terms of survival, a more important assessment of benefit than reperfusion, no time dependency was noted in the AIMS mortality study following anistreplase.[16]

The frequency of reperfusion was also dependent on the initial coronary flow grade. Anistreplase patients with an initial grade 1 flow showed reperfusion in 78% (21/27) cases, as opposed to 43% (38/88) of cases with an initial occlusion of grade 0. A similar result was obtained following intracoronary streptokinase therapy with reperfusion occurring in 77% (24/31) of patients with initial grade 1 flow and 54% (43/80) of patients with initial grade 0 flow.

Similar results were obtained in the Dutch reperfusion study[13] which compared intravenous anistreplase and intracoronary streptokinase (250,000 U) in patients treated within 4 hours of the onset of symptoms. Reperfusion was achieved in 64% (23/36) of patients treated with anistreplase and 67% (25/37) treated with intracoronary streptokinase. All were angiographically evaluated at 15 minute intervals up to 90 min post treatment. The mean time to reperfusion following anistreplase was about 45 min after the start of therapy.

It can be seen that, for those patients treated within 4 hours of the onset of symptoms, intravenous anistreplase therapy offers a similar reperfusion incidence to that obtained with intracoronary streptokinase. These rates are very similar to those obtained following administration of t-PA to patients within 4 hours of symptom onset.[14]

Patency

'Patency' studies differed from the above reperfusion studies in that pre-treatment coronary angiograms were not performed. Occlusion of the coronary arteries was inferred from clinical signs and symptoms and electrocardiographic evidence of AMI even after the administration of nitrates.

Hence for these studies the frequency of vessel patency following treatment rather than reperfusion is quoted. Patency of the infarct related artery in the first few hours after treatment was established by means of post-treatment angiography. Patency rates are commonly 10–20% higher than reperfusion rates since the coronary arteries may have reperfused spontaneously by the time treatment is administered and, in a small number of patients, myocardial infarction is not associated with occluding coronary arterial thrombi. These categories of patients would have been excluded in a reperfusion study in which pre-treatment angiograms were performed.

Two comparative studies were undertaken in patients with AMI in which the efficacy of anistreplase (30 U intravenous) injected over 2 to 5 minutes, was compared with intravenous streptokinase (1.5 million IU) infused over 60 minutes. Other uncontrolled studies were performed in which anistreplase was given to all patients. The prime objective of these studies was to assess the patency of the infarct related coronary artery angiographically.

One hundred and sixteen patients with AMI who had symptoms of less than 6 hour duration were enrolled into the larger of the two comparative studies with streptokinase.[17] The early patency rate (TIMI grades 2 and 3) assessed at a mean of 90 minutes after treatment was significantly different ($p < 0.05$) in the two groups: 70% for anistreplase treated patients and 51% for streptokinase treated patients. There were no significant differences in infarct site, or the time from treatment to angiography.

A smaller study, performed in Portugal and Spain, comparing the same treatment regimens also demonstrated that anistreplase therapy was associated with a significantly higher ($p = 0.02$) early patency rate than an intravenous infusion of streptokinase.[18] As in the previous study patients were stratified by site of infarction (anterior or inferior) before randomization to receive anistreplase ($n = 20$) or streptokinase ($n = 24$). Early patency was assessed by coronary angiography at a mean of 90 minutes after the start of treatment. TIMI grades 2 and 3 were considered as patent and were seen in 90% (18/20) anistreplase treated patients and 58% (14/24) streptokinase treated patients at this time interval ($p = 0.02$).

Other non-comparative studies have verified the high early patency rate observed after anistreplase therapy, giving results ranging from 70% to 100%.[19–21] A summary of the findings from patency and reperfusion studies involving anistreplase is given in Figure 2.

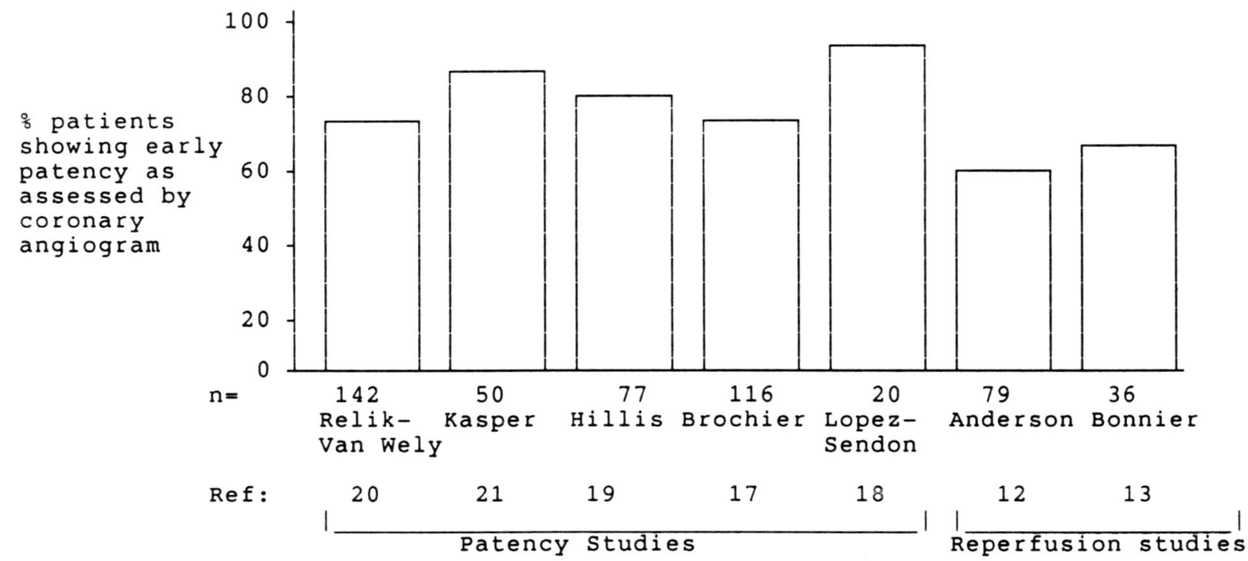

Figure 2 *Summary of patency and reperfusion studies*

Early reocclusion/reinfarction

Reperfusion of an infarct related vascular bed may be of little value if it is transient or persists only as long as the thrombolytic agent is present. It is therefore important to establish the incidence of early reocclusion, documented angiographically, or reinfarction based on clinical, electrocardiograhic or laboratory criteria.

Reocclusion was assessed angiographically within 24 hours of treatment in a number of studies. Anistreplase reocclusion rates were low in both the US and Dutch reperfusion studies, which compared anistreplase with intracoronary streptokinase.[12, 13] In the Dutch study,[13] the reocclusion rate was 5% (1/22) with anistreplase and 13% (3/23) with intracoronary streptokinase. The US study,[12] gave rates of 8% (3/40) for anistreplase and 3% (1/37) for intracoronary streptokinase.

A further Dutch study (open, involving 157 patients) investigated reocclusion rates at 24 hours after treatment following patency assessed at 90 minutes.[20] Of 103 patients evaluable by coronary angiography at 24 hours only 4 were found to have infarct related vessels that were not patent, i.e. a reocclusion rate of 4% at 24 hours following anistreplase.

The low reocclusion rates mentioned above are consistent with observations from the whole anistreplase clinical programme in which the incidence of reocclusion, assessed angiographically, and reinfarction within three days of anistreplase treatment, have been 4.5% (8/175) and 3.7% (39/1058) respectively.[22]

The anistreplase clinical programme was not designed to assess the efficacy of additional post-thrombolytic therapy or mechanical intervention. Anticoagulation with intravenous heparin was initiated 3–6 hours after thrombolytic therapy in most patients and continued for variable periods. In many studies, patients received oral anticoagulation – usually with warfarin for periods of up to 3 months. The use of other drug therapy such as aspirin was left to the discretion of the individual investigator. Clearly the use of such additional therapies may have had some effect on the reocclusion rates observed, but will have been similar in both anistreplase and control groups.

Myocardial salvage

One aim of thrombolysis in AMI is to improve morbidity by preservation of ventricular function.

Although there is now convincing evidence that thrombolytic therapy results in the lysis of thrombi responsible for occluding infarct-related coronary arteries, evidence for improvement in left ventricular function is more equivocal. Patel and Kloner[23] reviewed trials with streptokinase in AMI and found that an increase in ejection fraction was documented only in 2/7 intracoronary streptokinase trials and 1/2 intravenous streptokinase trials. In the anistreplase clinical programme, left ventricular function has been assessed by both radionuclide and contrast ventriculography in a number of studies.

In one multicentre, randomized, double-blind investigation of anistreplase (n = 112) in comparison with heparin (n = 119),[24] left ventricular ejection fraction (LVEF) was studied using both these methods.

Improved myocardial salvage amongst anistreplase-treated patients was demonstrated by significant preservation of ventricular function, as assessed by LVEF. Within the first week post-MI LVEF (determined from contrast angiography) was significantly higher in the anistreplase group than in the heparin group (p = 0.002). The benefit for patients treated with anistreplase

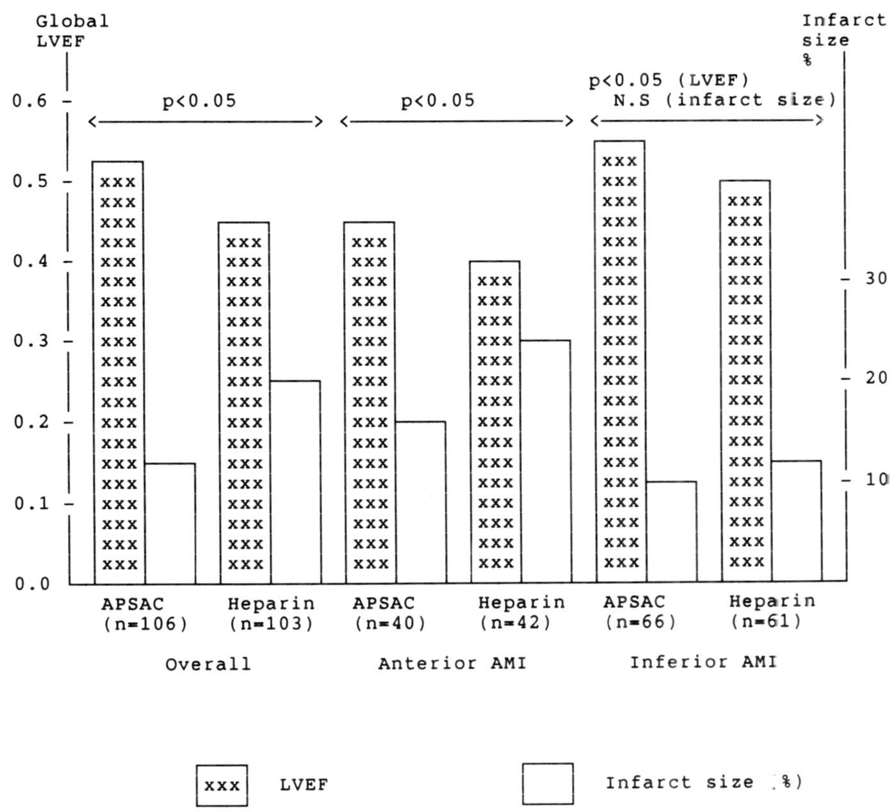

Figure 3 *Global LVEF and infarct size following anistreplase or heparin therapy by site of infarction* (after Bassand *et al.*, Ref. 24)

was found in both anterior (48% vs 40%, $p = 0.04$) and inferior (56% vs 52%, $p = 0.02$) myocardial infarctions (Fig. 3). LVEF was assessed further at about 3 weeks after treatment by radionuclide ventriculography. The difference between treatments, observed during the first week by contrast angiography, remained significant for the whole group ($p = 0.04$) at this assessment.

Infarct size was assessed in this study[24] by means of thallium-201 single photon emission computed tomography (SPECT) during the third week following myocardial infarction. The size of the infarct was, on average, 31% less in anistreplase-treated than in heparin-treated patients. This finding that anistreplase limits the size of infarction in comparison to conventional non-thrombolytic therapy was statistically significant ($p<0.01$) (Fig. 3). A close inverse relationship was found between the values of LVEF and infarct size ($r = -0.73$; $p<0.01$). It was concluded that anistreplase produced a significant reduction in infarct size which, in turn, resulted in significant preservation of left ventricular systolic function.

Results supportive to this finding come from an open comparative study[25] in which anistreplase ($n = 76$) was compared with a control group ($n = 73$) that received only standard non-thrombolytic therapy. In this study infarct size was assessed indirectly by measuring the R-wave score in the vulnerable chest leads at the time of discharge. The R-wave score was higher in the patients treated with anistreplase compared with controls and this effect was most marked in those treated within the first 2.5 hours of the onset of symptoms. These data indicate that the size of the myocardial infarction was less extensive in the group that received anistreplase than in those receiving control therapies.

The results of other studies in which left ventricular function was assessed are not so clear cut. However, similar inconsistencies have also been noted for streptokinase and may reflect methodological difficulties in demonstrating benefit rather than an absence of benefit in this regard. For example in a German study,[26] LVEF assessed prior to discharge from hospital was found to be similar in both anistreplase and heparin treatment groups. It is known that low LVEF is a predictor of early mortality following AMI. Anistreplase produced a 56% reduction in 28-day mortality compared with the placebo group in this study, so more patients with low LVEF were 'lost' from the heparin group than from the anistreplase group. Hence the similar LVEF values in the third week post-MI observed in both treatment groups can be interpreted as a positive result for anistreplase.

Mortality

The ultimate goal of thrombolytic therapy in acute myocardial infarction must be to improve survival. In the anistreplase programme, a number of studies have been undertaken in which mortality has been assessed in AMI patients following treatment with anistreplase or a non-thrombolytic comparator: placebo, heparin, or standard therapy. Principal among these was the APSAC intervention mortality study (AIMS)[16,27].

In this double-blind study, patients aged 70 years or less were randomized to anistreplase or placebo if they had symptoms lasting at least thirty minutes suggestive of acute myocardial infarction within the previous six hours. ECG evidence of ST segment elevation was required and patients were excluded if they were considered to be at risk of bleeding or had other contra-indications such as cardiogenic shock, severe hypertension, or concomitant anticoagulation therapy. Other treatments were not controlled except that all patients were given intravenous heparin, starting six hours after study treatment, followed by warfarin which was continued for at least six months, and timolol unless contraindicated.

An interim analysis was performed after 1000 patients had entered the study. This revealed that 61 (12.2%) of the patients receiving placebo, and 32 (6.4%) of those receiving anistreplase

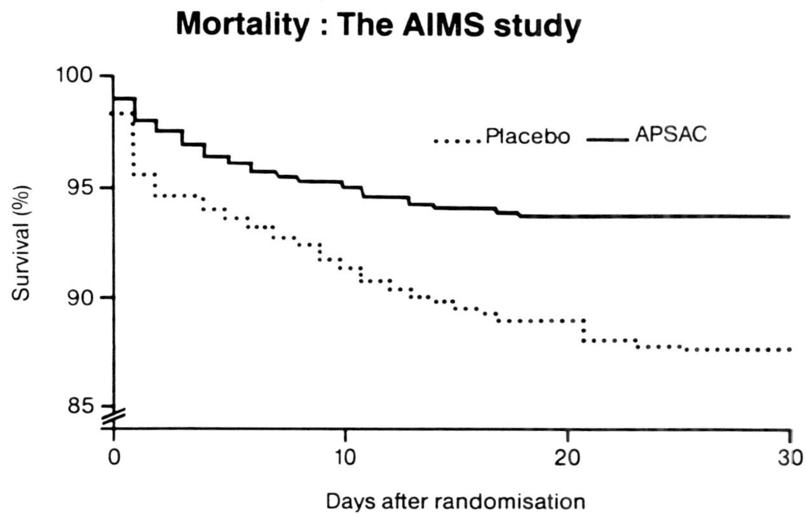

Figure 4 *30-day survival rates from the APSAC Intervention Mortality Study: complete data (n = 1251). Fox K A A (on behalf of The AIMS Trial Study Group) 1988, 10th Congress of Eur.Soc.Cardiol, Vienna (Symposium).*

Table 1 *Influence of individual variables in the APSAC intervention mortality study–sub-group analysis of 30-day mortality*

	30-day survival	
Variable	*Change in mortality hazard*	*Significance*
Treatment (*Anistreplase* vs Placebo)	− 55%	$p \leq 0.001$
Age (*under* 65 vs over 65 years)	− 72%	$p < 0.001$
Systolic BP (<*100* vs >100mm Hg)	+ 242%	$p < 0.001$
Heart rate (>*100* vs <80/mm)	+ 119%	$p = 0.005$
Previous MI (*Yes* vs no)	+ 79%	$p = 0.006$
Anterior vs inferior myocardial infarction	+ 157%	$p < 0.001$

[After Fox K A A (on behalf of the AIMS trial study group) 1988 10th Cong. Eur. Soc. Cardiol., Vienna] had died within 30 days of treatment (Fig. 4). From these figures, the estimated one year mortality was calculated to be 19.4% for placebo treated patients and 10.8% for anistreplase treated patients ($p = 0.0006$). This highly significant finding of a 47% reduction in 30 day mortality (($p = 0.0016$) 95% confidence interval: 21–65%) was sufficient evidence for the benefit of anistreplase in reducing mortality to terminate patient entry into the study. The independent data monitoring committee, responsible for ensuring that patients were not adversely affected by being given or denied therapy, felt it would be unethical to continue to randomize patients to a placebo treatment group.

Surprisingly, there was no evidence that early administration of anistreplase (i.e. within four hours of the onset of symptoms) caused any greater percentage reduction in mortality than later administration from four to six hours. However, there was a substantially higher mortality rate in the placebo group in the latter time category being 17.6% at thirty days compared with 9.2% in those treated within 0–4 hours.

Anistreplase decreased 30-day mortality in all subsets of patients evaluated (infarction site; MI history; age <65 or $\geqslant 65$ years; heart failure; gender; time since onset of symptoms, 0–4 hours or 4–6 hours). A proportional hazards model was used to assess simultaneously the influence of some individual variables on 30-day mortality (Table 1).

Independently, anistreplase treatment, age, systolic blood pressure, heart rate, previous myocardial infarction, and site of infarction all had highly significant effects on mortality. The beneficial effect of anistreplase appeared to be both proportionately and absolutely greater in patients aged over 65. Over 65s were a group found to be associated with a particularly high 30-day mortality – 30.2% in those allocated placebo, reduced to 12.2% in those treated with anistreplase.

Very few patients in this study received aspirin. Any additional beneficial effect on mortality due to combining anistreplase and aspirin awaits evaluation.

The AIMS study provides the strongest evidence in support of the claim that anistreplase has a significant effect on improving survival when administered in the first few hours following the onset of acute myocardial infarction.

Similar mortality results were obtained from a smaller randomized, controlled trial conducted in Germany[26] which compared anistreplase with heparin. In that study patients were randomized following MI of less than 4 hours' duration.

Survival within the first 28 days after MI was significantly higher in the anistreplase group, ($p = 0.03$). Nine deaths (5.6%) occurred in the anistreplase group and 19 (12.6%) in the heparin group, i.e. a 55.8% reduction in 28-day mortality in the anistreplase group in comparison to the heparin group (95% confidence limits, 5.4%–79.4%).

Pooled data from all clinical studies conducted with anistreplase indicate that mortality within 30 days of treatment has been 239/3850 (6.2%) in the anistreplase group, compared with 137/1244 (11.0%) in those who received non-thrombolytic therapy. The overall mortality any time after treatment has been 288/3850 (7.5%) and 171/1244 (13.7%) in the two treatment groups respectively.

Safety and tolerance

Data are available on over 5000 patients who have been recruited into the anistreplase clinical programme. Of these, 3850 patients have received anistreplase, 319 have received streptokinase and 1244 have received non-thrombolytic therapy (heparin, placebo or conventional therapy).

The vast majority of the anistreplase-treated patients received the standard dose of 30 Units injected over 2 to 5 minutes within 6 hours of symptom onset (the mean time to treatment being about 3 hours). This review presents the pooled safety data from all studies. Where appropriate the data are presented by study type. Incidence figures quoted refer to all adverse events recorded, regardless of clinical significance or possible relationship to therapy, in closely monitored studies.

The population of patients included in the studies appears to be similar to the AMI population at large, being predominantly male, middle-aged, about one-third having a history of angina and/or hypertension, a minority (approximately 10–24%) having a history of previous AMI, and about equal proportions of patients with anterior and inferior (right and circumflex coronary artery) lesions.

Cardiovascular events

Arrhythmias and conduction disorders were the most frequently occurring cardiovascular events and were reported in 1624/3850 (42%) of those who received anistreplase compared to 567/1244 (46%) of those who received non-thrombolytic therapy in all types of study. This latter group of patients received either placebo (as in the AIMS study), a bolus dose of heparin (as in the German EMS), or standard control therapy. Both groups of patients usually received infusion of heparin, which in the anistreplase group started 3–6 hours after treatment. The incidence of arrhythmias/conduction disorders in non-invasive studies was approximately twice that in invasive studies (51.4% vs 24.6% respectively). This difference possibly arises because the non-invasive studies usually included, as part of the clinical assessment, a specific question regarding reperfusion arrhythmias, resulting in a higher reporting incidence. In comparative invasive studies information on reperfusion arrhythmias was not specifically sought and the period of follow-up was relatively short, often 2–5 days. As a result the incidence of events reported was substantially lower – 71/289 (25%) following anistreplase, and 69/260 (27%) following streptokinase therapy.

In a double-blind, placebo-controlled mortality study (AIMS) the overall incidence of all arrhythmias was similar between the treatment groups. However, in the first 24 hours after dosing there was a higher incidence of idioventricular rhythm, ventricular extrasystoles, and ventricular tachycardia in the anistreplase group compared with placebo – a finding consistent with the higher incidence of reperfusion in the anistreplase group. These arrhythmias are

Table 2 *Incidence and aetiology of CVA occurring within 7 days of treatment*

*Aetiology**	*Anistreplase (n = 4391)*	*Non-thrombolytic (n = 1262)*
Haemorrhagic	18	0
Non-haemorrhagic	8	2
Unknown	10	2
Total of possible haemorrhagic**	28 (0.64%)	2 (0.16%)
Overall total	36 (0.82%)	4 (0.32%)

* Aetiology usually based on findings of CAT scan or post-mortem.
** Includes those of haemorrhagic and unknown aetiology.

relatively benign. Of those arrhythmias/conduction disorders reported, only ventricular fibrillation and cardiac arrest are likely to be immediately life-threatening. The incidences of those events were lower following anistreplase than following placebo treatment. The numbers of patients in the anistreplase and placebo groups with ventricular fibrillation within the first 24 hours of therapy were 15/500 and 20/501 respectively, and at any time in-hospital were 29/500 and 38/501 respectively. Cardiac arrest occurred within 24 hours of therapy in 11/500 anistreplase-treated and 14 placebo-treated patients, and at any time during the in-hospital period in 24/500 and 43/501 anistreplase or placebo patients respectively.

The incidence of hypotension (defined by a decrease of greater than 10 mmHg in either systolic or diastolic pressure (within 1 hour of dosing) and a systolic of less than 100 mmHg or diastolic of less than 60 mmHg, either reported as an adverse event by the investigator or where a low blood pressure recording was noted on the case record form, was 11% (434/3850) following anistreplase, 13% (42/319) following streptokinase and 8% (99/1244) following non-thrombolytic therapy: a slight excess (3%) in the anistreplase group compared with the non-thrombolytic.

Almost all patients received other vaso-active medications, such as nitrates and narcotic analgesics, and it is difficult to separate the possible hypotensive effects of these agents from that induced by thrombolytic therapy. Hypotension, however, has been reported to occur in conjunction with reperfusion (Bezold-Jarisch reflex)[28] and the increased incidence of hypotension following anistreplase treatment may reflect the increased reperfusion rates with thrombolytic therapy.

Within the anistreplase group the incidence of hypotension was lower in non-invasive studies than in invasive studies, 10% and 18% respectively. The administration of contrast dye to anistreplase-treated patients in invasive studies, together with the catheterization procedure itself, may contribute to the increased incidence of hypotension in this group.

High rates of streptokinase infusion have been reported to be associated with an increased incidence of hypotension.[29] Therefore the relationship of blood pressure to rate of injection has been examined for anistreplase patients where anistreplase was administered within the range 2 to 5 minutes. No relationship was noted between duration of anistreplase injection within this range and incidence of decrease in blood pressure. [Beecham data on file].

In keeping with the fact that anistreplase improves LVF, there was a lower incidence of heart failure in the anistreplase group than the non-thrombolytic – 8% versus 17%.

Cerebrovascular accidents

Cerebrovascular accidents (CVA) occurring at any time after therapy have been reported in 52/4391 (1.2%) patients in the anistreplase group and in 10/1262 (0.8%) patients in the non-thrombolytic group. Of these, the incidence of possible haemorrhagic CVA – which includes those definitely considered haemorrhagic and those of unknown aetiology – was 0.82% in the anistreplase group and 0.47% in the non-thrombolytic group.

The incidence of a CVA which is of haemorrhagic or unknown origin within 7 days of treatment with a thrombolytic is similar following anistreplase treatment (0.64%) or streptokinase treatment (0.61%) and is not significantly higher than that following non-thrombolytic therapy (0.16%) – an excess incidence of 0.5% (Table 2). Most patients in all three treatment groups received concomitant heparin and this undoubtedly may have some effect on the CVA incidence recorded.

In the majority of these cases, predisposing conditions, such as hypertension, previous CVA, or surgical intervention, may have placed those patients at greater risk of developing a CVA.

Haemorrhagic events

Haemorrhagic events were reported in 644/3850 (16.7%) of those who received anistreplase. The majority of these were minor events, the most frequent being puncture site haemorrhage or haematoma which occurred in 6.8% (264/3850) of patients, the majority of which were in invasive studies. Only in 1.9% of anistreplase treated patients (72/3850) were the haemorrhagic events described as severe by the investigator. The incidences of severe haemorrhagic events following streptokinase and non-thrombolytic therapy were 3.1% (10/323) and 0.4% (5/1244) respectively.

Bleeding events other than at puncture sites occurred in 11.5% (446/3850) of anistreplase treated patients. Haematuria, anaemia, GI bleeding and bruising accounted for approximately 90% of these other events. Bleeding at other sites was reported infrequently.

Not surprisingly the incidence of haemorrhagic events was higher in the invasive than the non-invasive studies, 22% versus 13% (64/289 and 163/1246 respectively). This difference was due to a higher incidence of puncture site haemorrhages in the invasive studies, 14.5%, versus 4.9% in non-invasive (42/289 and 62/1246 respectively). The occurrence of puncture site bleeding is higher in invasive studies as frequently arterial catheterization was required. The incidence of bleeding events other than puncture site haemorrhages was similar in the two groups of studies. In studies in which anistreplase and intravenous streptokinase were compared the incidence of haemorrhagic events was similar and was in turn higher than in non-thrombolytic control patients.

It appears that treatment with thrombolytics can increase the risk of bleeding by about 10–11 percentage points but that non-thrombolytic therapy (which includes treatment with heparin alone) also has associated with it a small bleeding risk (about 3.8% incidence). The apparent risk of bleeding following anistreplase therapy is complicated by the fact that most patients were also treated with some anticoagulant and so the risk of bleeding is not necessarily in consequence of anistreplase but for a treatment regimen which includes both anistreplase and anticoagulant.

Although no studies have examined specifically the effect of adding anti-platelet therapy to anistreplase, many of the patients involved in anistreplase studies received such agents, mostly aspirin at a mean dose of 200*mg/day.

The relative increase in incidence of haemorrhagic events observed when anti-platelet therapy was added to anistreplase was similar to the relative increase noted when it is added to non-thrombolytic therapy. The risk ratio comparing the incidences of haemorrhagic events reported with and without anti-platelet therapy was 1.41% for Eminase and 1.77% for non-thrombolytic therapy.

Possible 'allergic' reactions

Since the anistreplase complex contains streptokinase, a non-human protein, it is by its nature potentially allergenic. In practice, however, the incidence of clinically significant allergic events following anistreplase has been low. A similar finding has been reported for streptokinase.[30,31]

The overall incidence of all possible allergic-type reactions following anistreplase therapy (including allergic reactions, anaphylactoid reactions, angioedema, asthma, eosinophilia, pruritus and rash) was 0.8% for events occurring within 2 hours of therapy and 2.9% at any time following therapy. However, only 0.4% of these – approximately 15 patients – were considered severe by the investigator. The term 'possible allergic reaction' is used since in many cases there was no evidence that the event was allergic in aetiology.

In the double-blind placebo-controlled mortality trial (AIMS) the incidence of possible 'allergic-type' events was 3.0% in the anistreplase group and 2.4% in the placebo group.

The incidence of anaphylactoid reactions, perhaps the most severe form of allergic response, was low – 0.23% (8/3850) in the anistreplase treated group compared to 0.31% (1/323) in the streptokinase treated group. There were none reported following non-thrombolytic therapy. The term 'anaphylactoid reaction' has been used uncritically and includes all events described by the investigator as anaphylaxis, anaphylactic shock, and similar terms. A review of the available data would suggest, as did that from ISIS-2,[31] that these terms were often used inappropriately.

The number of reactions was too low to permit an analysis of the data to determine whether pre-treatment with antihistamines or steroids would reduce the incidence.

Vasculitis/purpuric rash similar to that reported for streptokinase has been noted in 14/3850 (0.36%) patients. In the majority of cases the purpuric rash was first observed 7–15 days after treatment with Eminase and was associated with other systemic events such as arthralgia and haematuria.[32] Patients recovered spontaneously without any sequelae.

Fever and chills have been reported with a similar incidence in all treatment groups (anistreplase 3.9%, streptokinase 3.7%, non-thrombolytics 3.5%).

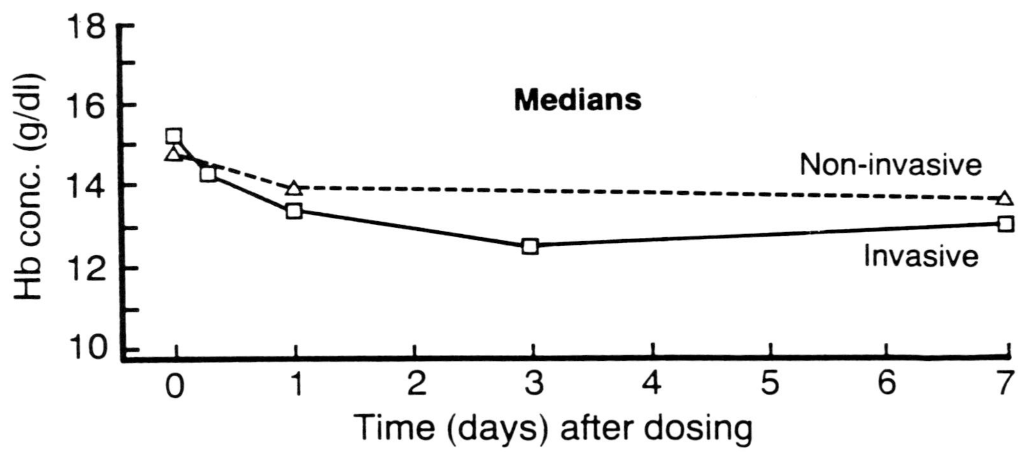

Figure 5 *Changes in haemoglobin concentration. Comparison of invasive and non-invasive studies* (APSAC)

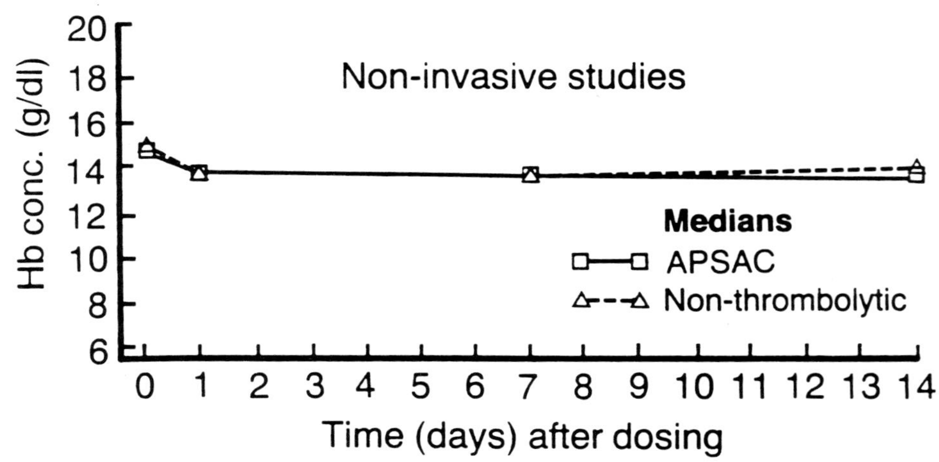

Figure 6 *Changes in haemoglobin concentration*

Other adverse events

Other adverse events have been reported following anistreplase treatment but the incidences of these have been similar to, or less than, those reported in the non-thrombolytic control group.

Effect on haemoglobin

As may be expected, larger falls in haemoglobin concentrations have been noted following anistreplase treatment in invasive than in non-invasive studies with peak falls of 2.5 g/dl and

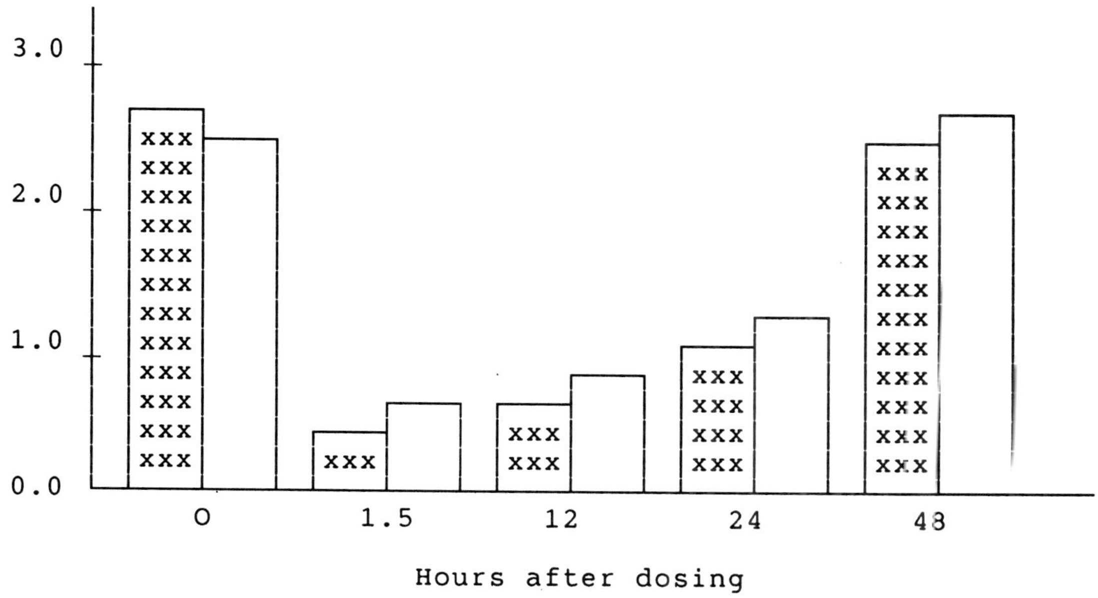

Figure 7 *Effect of intravenous anistreplase and intracoronary streptokinase on mean plasma fibrinogen levels* [33]

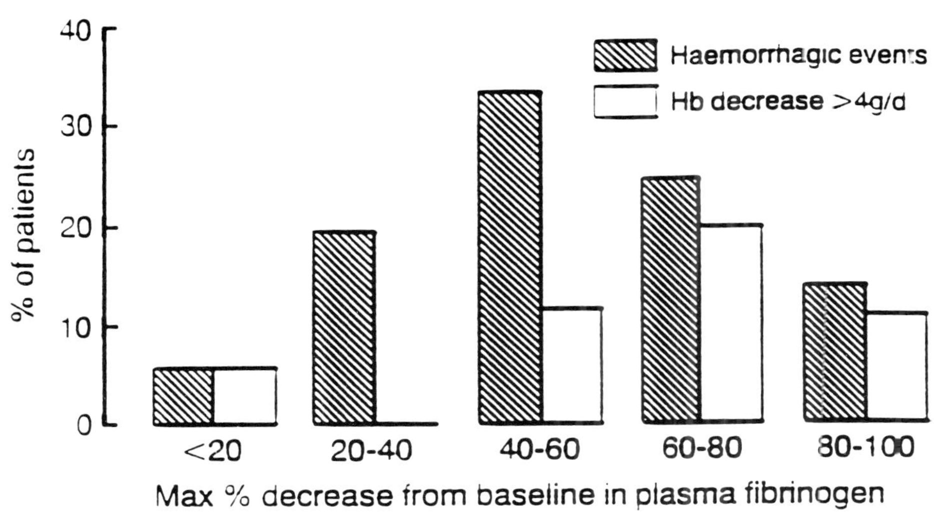

Figure 8 *Correlation of decreases in fibrinogen with haemorrhagic events and decreases in haemoglobin*

1.5 g/dl at 3 and 7 days respectively (Fig. 5). In the non-invasive studies, however, the falls in haemoglobin were similar following anistreplase or non-thrombolytic therapy (Fig. 6).

Falls in haemoglobin concentration may be used as an indirect measure of blood loss but other factors are also relevant here. For example, haemodilution resulting from a reversal of an initial vasoconstriction and consequent impaired haemodynamics with secondary fluid retention can account for some of the fall, especially in this population. Reduced serum protein concentrations, consistent with haemodilution, have been observed.

In terms of falls in haemoglobin greater than 4 g/dl (a figure many would associate with evidence of a major bleed) in the non-invasive studies, similar numbers of anistreplase and non-thrombolytic treated patients were noted (3.5% and 3.7% respectively).

Effect on blood clotting mechanism

Clinical studies which have measured clotting parameters have all demonstrated that treatment with anistreplase can produce a lytic state and systemic fibrinogenolysis.[21, 33, 34, 35] There were decreases in fibrinogen, plasminogen, factors II, V and VIII, α_2-antiplasmin, and increases in fibrin degradation products, i.e. thrombin time, activated partial thromboplastin time and pro-thrombin time.

In the Dutch reperfusion study[33] there were similar changes in fibrinogen levels following anistreplase and streptokinase (Fig. 7). Trough levels were seen at 1.5 h after treatment with levels returning to baseline within 24–48 hours. These data are thought to reflect accurately the time course of changes in fibrinogen levels although the magnitude of the change may be exaggerated by methodological problems resulting from continuing fibrinogenolysis *in vitro*.

All thrombolytics currently available result in systemic fibrinogenolysis which has been of concern in treating patients. A lytic state may, however, be beneficial in acute myocardial infarct patients as reduced blood viscosity could improve micro-perfusion and thus limit irreversible myocardial damage. Additionally, there is no clear correlation between systemic fibrinogenolysis and haemorrhagic complications or falls in haemoglobin following anistreplase (Fig. 8). A similar finding has been noted for t-PA. In a double-blind comparison of t-PA and streptokinase, although t-PA induced systemic fibrinogenolysis that was substantially less than that induced by streptokinase, the frequency of haemorrhagic events (33% t-PA, 31% streptokinase) and associated transfusions (22% t-PA, 20% streptokinase) was comparable in both groups.[36]

Other laboratory parameters

Large increases in aspartate transaminase (AST), alanine transaminase (ALT) and creatine phosphokinase (CPK) were seen in all studies after all treatments including anistreplase. Such increases are expected in patients with acute myocardial infarction due to the release of enzymes from damaged myocardial cells.

Any changes seen in other haematological or biochemical laboratory parameters were similar in all treatment groups and were not modified by anistreplase therapy.

Conclusions

Anistreplase has been shown to be an effective thrombolytic agent in the treatment of patients following acute myocardial infarction, producing:

- significant and substantial improvement in survival (short and long term)
- significant beneficial effects on myocardial salvage

- reperfusion rates similar to those with intracoronary SK
- patency rates superior to those with intravenous SK
- low reocclusion rates
- comparable side effect profile to other thrombolytics

coupled with the benefit of being administered as a single injection over 2–5 minutes.

References

1. Smith R A G, Dupe R J, English P D, Green J; Fibrinolysis with acyl-enzymes; a new approach to thrombolytic therapy. *Nature 290*, 1981, 505–508.
2. Ferres H, Hibbs M, Smith R A G. Deacylation studies *in vitro* on anistreplase. *Drugs 33* 1987, (Supplement 3), 80–82.
3. Been M, de Bono D P, Muir A L, *et al.*, Clinical effects and kinetic properties of intravenous anistreplase – anisoylated plasminogen streptokinase activator complex (BRL 26921) in acute myocardial infarction. *Int. J. Cardiol. 11*, 1986, 53-61.
4. Doenecke P, Schwerdt H, Hellstern P *et al.*, Bolus injection of anisoylated plasminogen streptokinase activator complex (BRL 26921) – a new approach to intravenous thrombolytic treatment of acute myocardial infarction. *Klin. Wochenschr. 64*, 1986, 682–687.
5. Mentzer R L, Budzynski A Z, Sherry S, High-dose brief-duration intravenous infusion of streptokinase in acute myocardial infarction: description of effects in circulation. *Am. J. Cardiol. 57*, 1986, 1220–1226.
6. Fletcher A P, Alkjaersig N, Sherry S, *et al.*, The development of urokinase as a thrombolytic agent. Maintenance of sustained thrombolytic state in man by its intravenous infusion. *J. Lab. Clin. Med. 65*, 1965, 713–731.
7. Van de Werf F, Nobuhara M, Collen D, Coronary thrombolysis with human single-chain, urokinase-type plasminogen activator (pro-urokinase) in patients with acute myocardial infarction. *Ann. Intern. Med. 104*, 1986, 345–349.
8. Verstraete M, Collen D, Thrombolytic therapy in the eighties. *Blood 67*, 1986, 1529–1541.
9. Marder V J, Rothbard R L, Fitzpatric P G, Francis C W, Norry E C, Dose ranging studies of Anisoylated Plasminogen Streptokinase Activator complex: Studies in healthy volunteers and in patients with acute myocardial infarction. *Drugs 33* (Supplement 3), 1987, 124–132.
10. Jackson D, Summary of early clinical experience with Anisoylated Plasminogen Streptokinase Activator complex in the treatment of acute myocardial infarction. *Drugs 33* (Supplement 3), 1987, 104–111.
11. Timmis A D, Griffin B, Crick J C P, Sowton E, Anisoylated plasminogen streptokinase activator complex in acute myocardial infarction: a placebo-controlled arteriographic coronary recanalization study. *J. Am. Coll. Cardiol. 10*, 1987, 205–210.
12. Anderson J L, Rothbard R L, Hackworthy R A, Sorenson S G, Fitzpatrick P G, Dahl C F, Hagan A D, Browne K F, Symkoviak G P, Menlove R L, Barry W H, Eckerson H W, Marder V J, for the anistreplase Multicenter Investigators. Multicenter reperfusion trial of intravenous anisoylated plasminogen streptokinase activator complex (anistreplase) in acute myocardial infarction: controlled comparison with intracoronary streptokinase. *J. Am. Coll. Cardiol. 11*, 1988, 1153–1156.
13. Bonnier J J R M, Vissier R F, Klomps H C, Hoffman H J M L and the Dutch Invasive Reperfusion Study Group. Comparison of intravenous anisoylated plasminogen streptokinase activator complex and intracoronary streptokinase in acute myocardial infarction. *Am. J. Cardiol. 62*, 1988, 25–30.
14. Chesebro J H, Knatterud G, Roberts R, *et al.*, Thrombolysis in Myocardial Infarction (TIMI) trial, Phase I: A comparison between intravenous tissue plasminogen activator and

intravenous streptokinase. *Circulation 76*, 1987, 142–154.
15. Verstraete M, Bernard R, Bory M, *et al.*, Randomised trial of intravenous recombinant tissue-type plasminogen activator versus intravenous streptokinase in acute myocardial infarction. Report from the European Co-operative Study Group for recombinant tissue-type plasminogen activator. *Lancet 1*, 1985, 842–847.
16. Fox K A A (on behalf of the AIMS Trial Study Group). The Anistreplase Intervention Mortality Study (AIMS). A placebo-controlled mortality trial of anistreplase in acute myocardial infarction: mortality results from the complete study. In *Eminase: Clinical benefits and survival of myocardial infarct patients treated with Eminase (anistreplase),* Chamberlain D A and Boissel J P (eds). An international symposium at the Xth Congress of the European Society of Cardiology, Vienna, 31st August 1988. Amsterdam, *Excerpta Medica*, 1988, 35–38.
17. Brochier M L on behalf of the Invasive Reperfusion Study II Group. Intravenous thrombolytic therapy with anistreplase in acute myocardial infarction. In *Eminase: Clinical benefits and survival of myocardial infarct patients treated with Eminase (anistreplase)*, Chamberlain D A and Boissel J P (eds). An international symposium at the Xth Congress of the European Society of Cardiology, Vienna, 31st August 1988. Amsterdam; *Excerpta Medica*, 1988, 8–9.
18. Lopez-Sendon J, Seabra-Gomes R, Martin Santos F, Calvo L, Silva J A, Macaya C, Munoz J, Miquel J, Sobrino N, Aleixo A, Gonzalez Maqueda I, Martin Jadraque L, La Paz H, Intravenous anisoylated plasminogen streptokinase activator complex (anistreplase) versus intravenous streptokinase (SK) in myocardial infarction (AMI). A randomised multicentre study. *Eur. Heart. J. 9* (Supplement 1), 1988, Abstract no. 73.
19. Hillis W S, Hornung R S, Hogg K J, Hockings N, Dunn F G, Achievement of coronary artery patency by use of anisoylated plasminogen streptokinase activator complex in acute myocardial infarction. *Drugs 33* (Supplement 3), 1987, 117–123.
20. Relik-van Wely L, Visser R F, van der Pol J M J, Vet A J T M, Drost H, Klomps H C, Berg F, Aarts F J E M, den Heyer P, van Dijk R B, Anistreplase reocclusion study at 24 hours. A preliminary report of the angiographically assessed patency and reocclusion in patients with an acute myocardial infarction (AMI) treated with anistreplase. A Dutch multicentre study. In *Eminase: Clinical benefits and survival of myocardial infarct patients treated with Eminase (anistreplase)*, Chamberlain D A and Boissel J P (eds). An international symposium at the Xth Congress of the European Society of Cardiology, Vienna, 31st August 1988. Amsterdam; *Excerpta Medica*, 1988, 10–14.
21. Kasper W, Meinertz T, Wollschläger H, *et al.*, Coronary thrombolysis during acute myocardial infarction by intravenous BRL 26921, a new anisoylated plasminogen streptokinase activator complex. *Am. J. Cardiol. 58*, 1986, 418–421.
22. Cregeen R J, Johnson E S, A review of the safety of Eminase. In *Eminase: Clinical benefits and survival of myocardial infarct patients treated with Eminase (anistreplase)*, Chamberlain D A and Boissel J P (eds). An international symposium at the Xth Congress of the European Society of Cardiology, Vienna, 31st August 1988. Amsterdam; *Excerpta Medica*, 1988, 42–43.
23. Patel B, Kloner R A, Analysis of reported randomised trials of streptokinase therapy for acute myocardial infarction in the 1980's. *Am. J. Cardiol. 59*, 1987, 501–504.
24. Bassand J P, Machecourt J, Cassagnes J, Anguenot T, Lusson R, Borel E, Peycelon P, Wolf E, Ducellier D, for the APSIM Study investigators. Multicentre trial of intravenous anisoylated plasminogen streptokinase activator complex (anistreplase) in acute myocardial infarction. Effects on infarct size and left ventricular function. *J. Am.Coll. Cardiol. 13*, 1989, 988–997.

25. Ikram S, Lewis G, Bucknall C, Sram I, Thomas N, Vincent R, Chamberlain D, Treatment of Acute myocardial infarction with anisoylated plasminogen streptokinase activator complex. *Br. Med. J. 293*, 1986, 786–789.
26. Meinertz T, Kasper W, Schumacher M, Just H, for the anistreplase Multicenter Trial Group. The German multicenter trial of anisoylated plasminogen streptokinase activator complex versus heparin for acute myocardial infarction. *Am. J. Cardiol. 62*, 1988, 347–351.
27. AIMS Trial Study Group. Effect of intravenous anistreplase on mortality after acute myocardial infarction: preliminary report of a placebo-controlled clinical trial. *Lancet 1*, 1988, 545–549.
28. Korern G, Weiss A T, Ben-David Y, Hasan Y, Luria H, Gotsman M S. Bradycardia and hypotension following reperfusion with streptokinase (Bezold-Jarisch reflex): A sign of coronary thrombolysis and myocardial salvage. *Am. Heart Journal 112*, 1986, 468–471.
29. Lews A S, *et al.* The hypotensive effect of intravenous streptokinase in patients with acute myocardial infarction. *Circulation 72*, 1985, 1321–1326.
30. Gruppo Italiano per lo Studio della Streptochinasi nell'Infarto miocardico (GISSI). Effectiveness of intravenous thrombolytic treatment in acute myocardial infarction. *Lancet 1*, 1986, 397–402.
31. ISIS-2 (Second International Study of Infarct Survival) Collaborative Group. Randomised trial of intravenous streptokinase, oral aspirin, both, or neither among 17, 187 cases of suspected acute myocardial infarction: ISIS-2. *Lancet 2*, 1988, 349–360.
32. Bucknall C, Darley, Flax J, Vincent R, Chamberlain D, Vasculitis complicating treatment with intravenous anisoylated plasminogen streptokinase activator complex in acute myocardial infarction. *Br.Heart J. 59*, 1988, 9–11.
33. Hoffmann J J M L, Bonnier J J R M, de Swart J B R M, Custers P, Vijgen M, Systemic effects of anistreplase and streptokinase therapy in acute myocardial infarction. Coagulation aspect of the Dutch Invasive Reperfusion Study. *Drugs 33* (Supplement 3), 1987, 242–246.
34. Marder V J, Kinsella P A, Brown M J, Fibrinogen concentration and coronary artery reperfusion after intravenous anistreplase or i.c. streptokinase therapy. *Drugs 33* (Supplement 3), 1987, 237–241.
35. Samama M, Conrad J, Verdy E, *et al.*, Biological study of intravenous anisoylated plasminogen streptokinase activator complex in acute myocardial infarction. *Drugs 33* (Supplement 3), 1987, 268–274.
36. Rao A K, Pratt C, Berke A, Jaffe A, Ockene I, Schreiber T L, Bell W R, Knatterud G, Robertson T L, Terrin M L, Thrombolysis in Myocardial Infarction (TIMI) Trial – Phase I: Haemorrhagic manifestations and changes in plasma fibrinogen and the fibrinolytic system in patients treated with recombinant tissue plasminogen activator and streptokinase. *J. Am. Coll. Cardiol. 11*, 1988, 1–11.

Chapter 4

MECHANISMS BY WHICH THROMBOLYSIS REDUCES MORTALITY: LIMITATION OF INFARCT SIZE – WHAT ELSE?

Rolf Schröder

Freie Universität, Berlin

The hypothesis underlying thrombolytic therapy for acute myocardial infarction is that reperfusion will salvage myocardium and thereby enhance survival. However, improved survival has also been demonstrated in patients in whom thrombolysis was initiated far too late to salvage relevant proportions of ischemic myocardium 'at risk'.[1]

Some studies have indicated improvement in left ventricular function and a lower mortality rate in patients in whom patency of the infarct-related vessel was achieved as compared with patients in whom the artery remained occluded, even when thrombolysis was performed relatively so late that actual salvage of myocardium was minimal.[2,3] However, whether and to what extent late patency of an infarct-related coronary artery is of benefit, is still a matter of debate.

In patients not given thrombolytic therapy definite improvement in left ventricular function in those with a patent infarct artery 1 month after myocardial infarction has also been documented. It is, however, unclear whether left ventricular improvement is due to early spontaneous reperfusion or to what extent it may also result from late reopening of the infarct artery.[4]

This report will deal mainly with results of the ISAM study and consists of two parts: first, the actual salvage of proportions of ischemic 'at risk' myocardium by timely reperfusion causing direct limitation of infarct size, and second, the potential additive impact of late reperfusion on left ventricular function: 'indirect' limitation of infarct size.

Method

The ISAM study was a double-blind placebo-controlled German-Swiss-Canadian multicenter study, carried out between March 1982 and March 1985. 1741 patients seen within 6 hours of onset of symptoms of myocardial infarction were randomly allocated to either 1.5 MU i.v. streptokinase or placebo infusion.[5,6] 12-lead ECGs were recorded before and 3 hours, 24 hours, 3 weeks and 7 months after randomization. Evolving myocardial infarction was diagnosed if typical symptoms and ST segment elevations were present, of at least 1 mm in one or more in limb leads or of at least 2 mm or more in the chest leads. MB-CK serum concentrations were determined every 2 hours for the first 30 hours and every 4 hours for the next 20 hours. Cardiac catheterization and angiography were performed 31 ± 12 days after myocardial infarction. Coronary arteriography and ventricular angiograms were obtained with contrast enhancement adequate for quantitative analysis in 52% of all patients alive after 21 days. Patients who had angiography were significantly younger than those who had no angiography (54.8 ± 9.5 vs 61.3 ± 9.4 y, $p<0.001$). Otherwise there was no difference in all other baseline variables including the ischemic area at risk, the ECG-infarct score or enzyme infarct size. There was no selection with regard to treatment with streptokinase or placebo.

Ischemic area at risk: The sum of ST-segment elevations in the pre-randomization ECG from leads I, aVL and V1–V6 for anterior myocardial infarction was defined as the ischemic area at risk. There was a highly significant linear relationship when the size of the ischemic area at risk was compared with the fully evolved ECG and enzymatic or angiographic infarct size. The magnitude of the sum of ST-segment elevations at baseline was also a strong prognosticator of short- and long-term mortality.[7]

ECG-infarct size was calculated by means of an QRS-Score: for the first part Σ R-amplitude (A-D) and for the second part Σ R-amplitude (A-D) + 10 × number of Q-waves (D-A). A = ECG on admission, D = ECG at 3 weeks (discharge). ECG leads were selected as representing the ischemic area at risk, depending on anterior or interior location of the infarct.

Enzyme infarct size was calculated from the area under the serum MB-CK time-activity curve with a zero line of 10 IU/1. Enzyme activity curves were plotted with three-point smoothing. The MB-CK area corresponds with the cumulative MB-CK release.

Ejection fraction was calculated from an angiogram in the 30° right anterior oblique projection according to the area length method. Regional abnormalities in the left ventricular wall motion were calculated in square units as the 'regional dyssynergic area' (regional DA). In brief, the end-diastolic and end-systolic silhouettes were divided into 48 segmental radii with equal angles. Shortening of segmental radii by less than 2 SD of the normal range for systolic shortening in healthy subjects was considered indicative of a dyssynergic radius. The dyssynergic area was calculated from the sum of dyssynergic radii. Only the areas involved in the infarction qualifying them for the study were evaluated.[5]

An infarct-related artery was judged patent if the residual diameter stenosis was 95% and there was complete perfusion, i.e. filling and clearance of contrast in the coronary bed distal to the stenosis as rapid as in other coronary beds (TIMI grade 3 perfusion).

It was stated prospectively that the results in patients treated within 3 hours should be compared with results in patients treated between 3 and 6 hours after the onset of symptoms.

Statistical analysis

Group differences were assessed by the two-sample *t* or chi-square test for continuous and dichotomous variables, respectively. Two-sided p-values are cited. All values are expressed as mean ± standard deviation of the mean.

Results

Actual limitation of infarct size

In Figures 1–12 are shown the actually developed ECG-infarct sizes (Figs 1–3) and MB-CK enzyme infarct sizes (Figs 4–6) as well as the global ejection fraction (Figs 7–9) and the regional wall motion abnormalities, i.e. the regional dyssynergic area (Figs 9–12) for the total groups of streptokinase and placebo treated patients, and for the subgroup of patients treated within 3 hours or between 3 and 6 hours of symptom onset. For the ECG infarct size and enzyme infarct size there was a significant difference in favor of streptokinase for the total group and for those treated within 3 hours of symptom onset. Patients treated within the first hour of symptom onset benefited most. In patients with inferior myocardial infarction a difference in favor of streptokinase could be demonstrated only for patients who were treated within the first hour. However, since inferior infarction QRS scores correspond poorly with enzyme infarct size, with regional ejection fraction from contrast angiograms or with pathological infarct sizes, QRS score is probably a poor measure for inferior infarcts.

Comparing anterior and inferior myocardial infarction, it is apparent that limitation of infarct size is significant in patients with anterior myocardial infarction treated within the first 4 hours, but only in those treated within the first 2 hours after symptom onset in patients with inferior myocardial infarction.

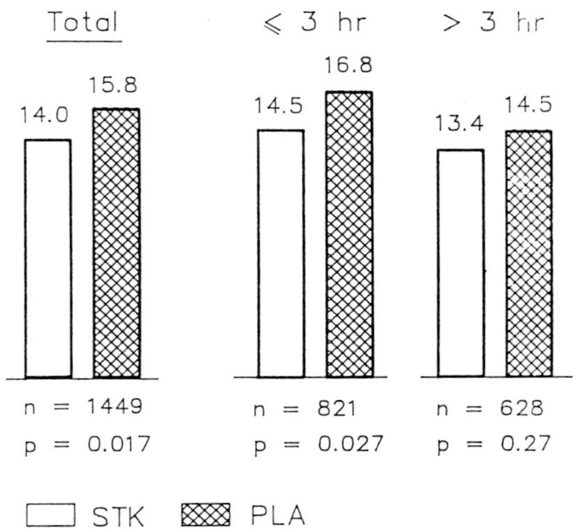

Figure 1 *ECG infarct size*

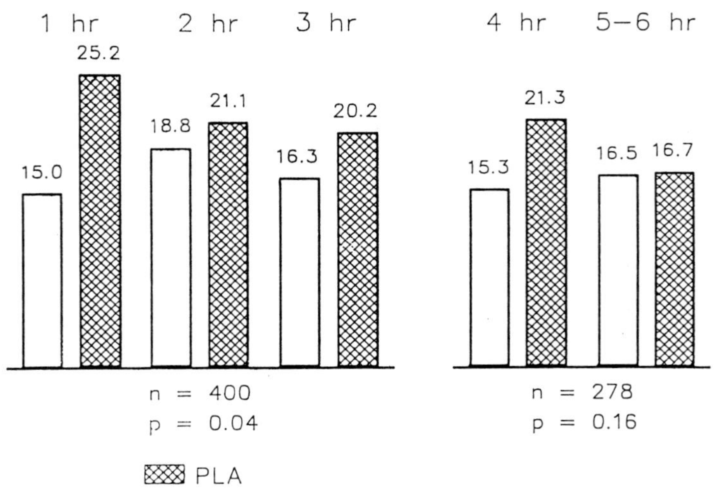

Figure 2 *ECG infarct size, anterior MI*

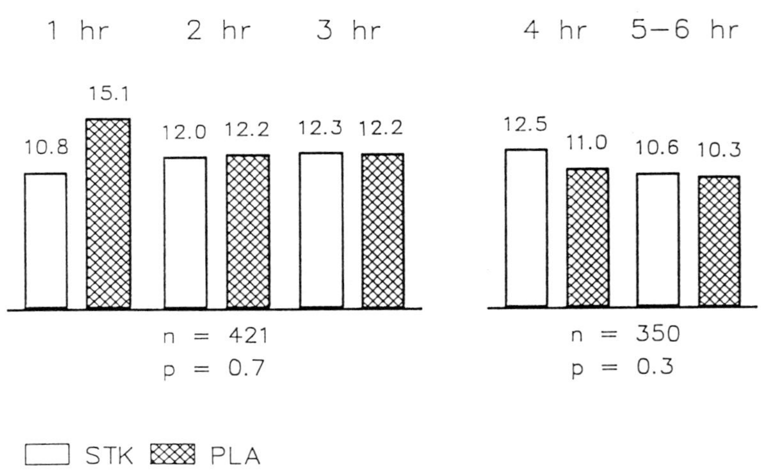

Figure 3 *ECG infarct size, inferior MI*

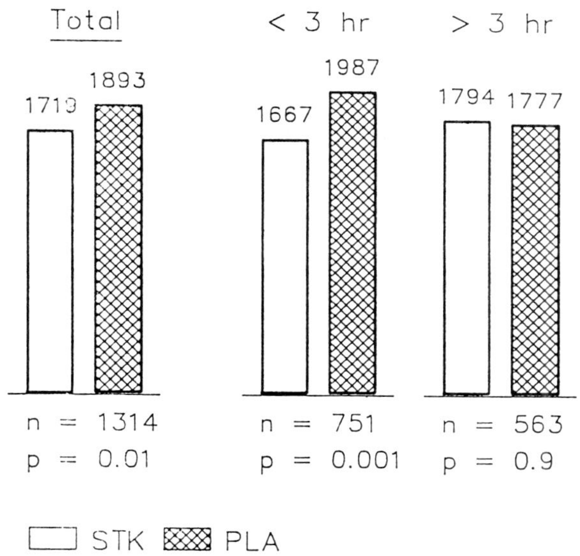

Figure 4 *Enzyme infarct size*

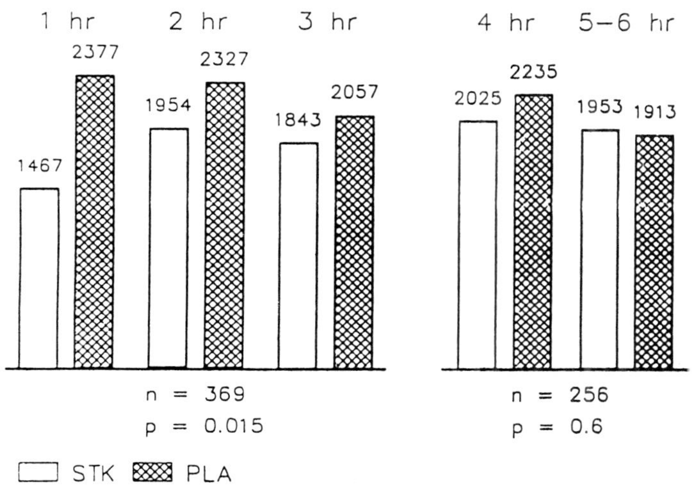

Figure 5 *Enzyme infarct size, anterior MI*

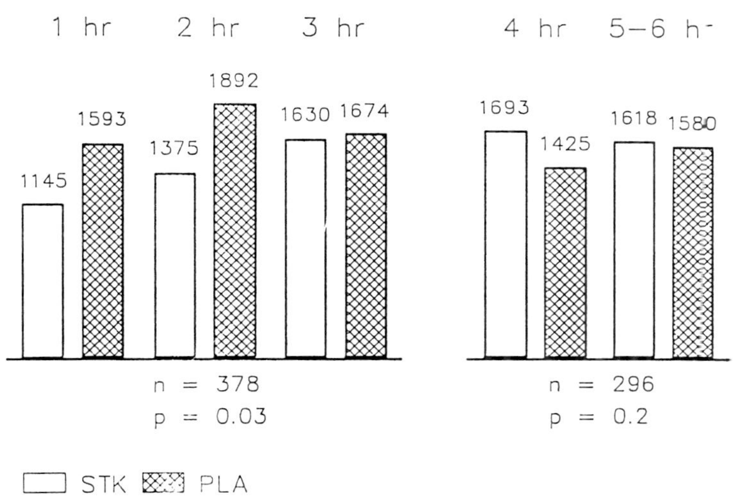

Figure 6 *Enzyme infarct size, inferior MI*

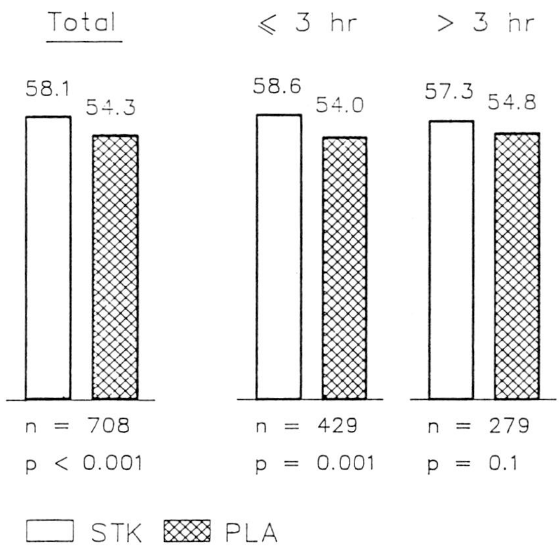

Figure 7 *Ejection fraction*

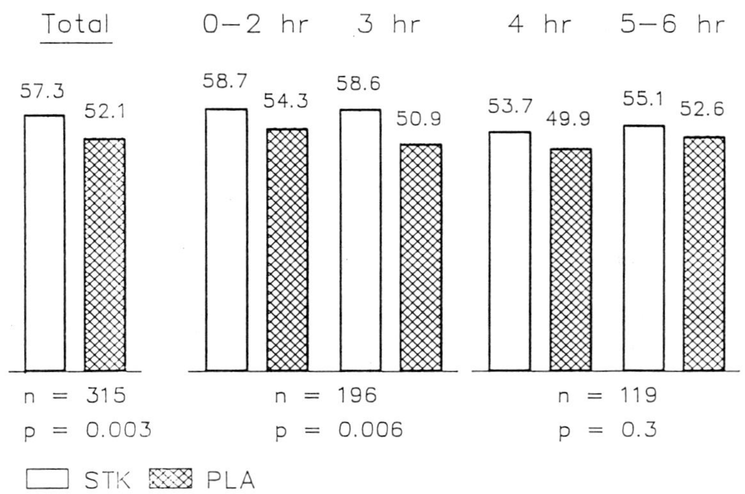

Figure 8 *Ejection fraction, anterior MI*

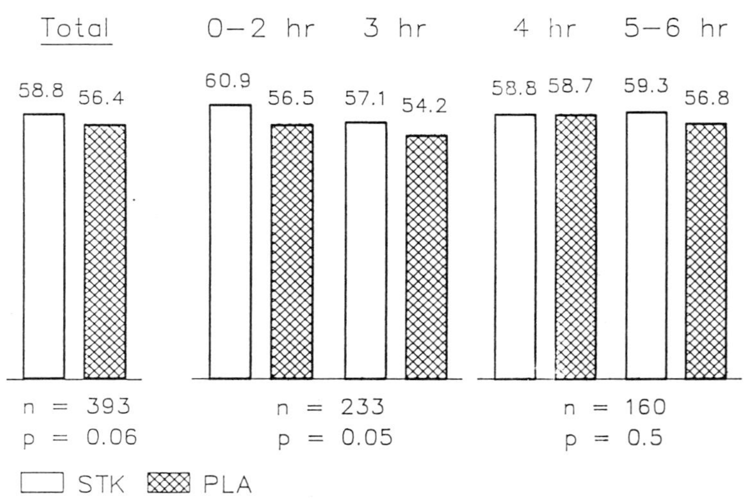

Figure 9 *Ejection fraction, inferior MI*

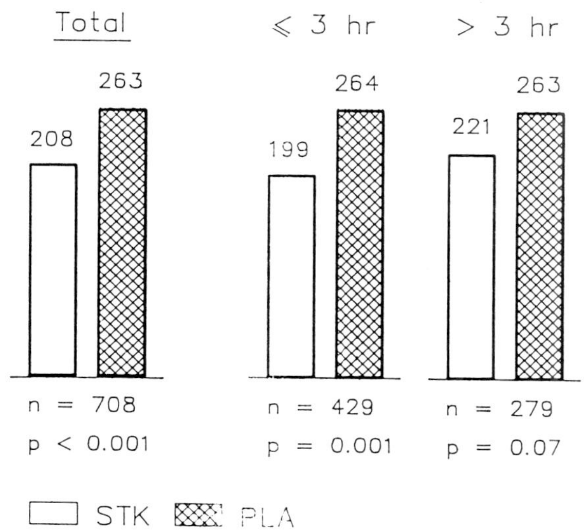

Figure 10 *Angio infarct size*

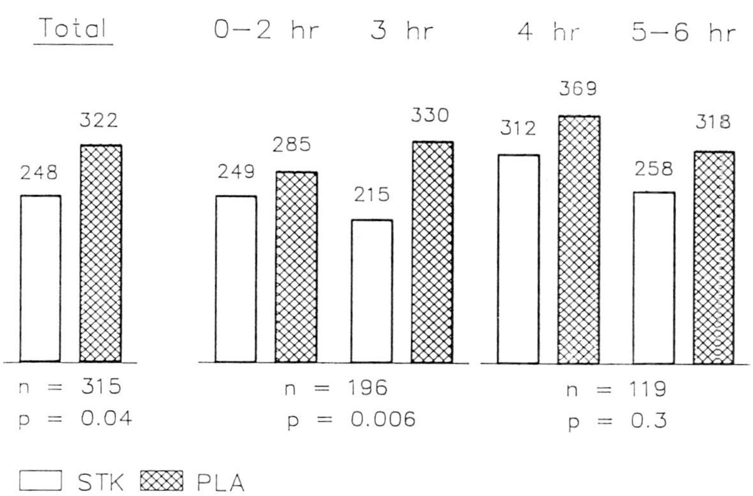

Figure 11 *Angio infarct size, anterior MI*

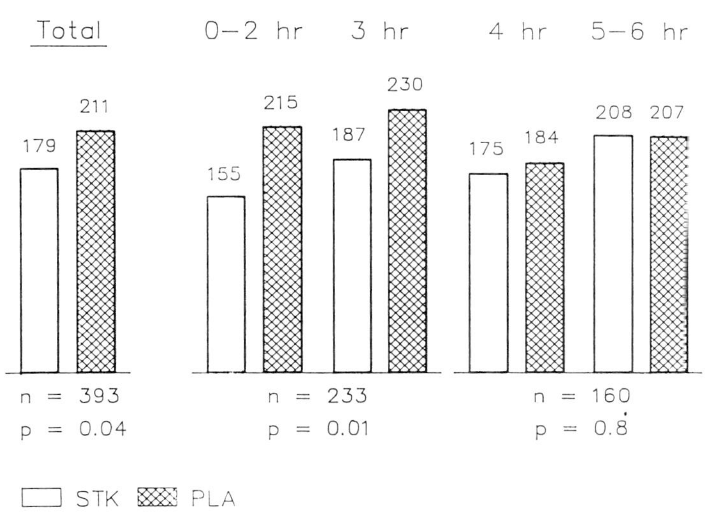

Figure 12 *Angio infarct size, inferior MI*

Global ejection fraction and regional dyssynergic area of the left ventricle were also significantly better in streptokinase treated patients as compared with placebo patients. Compared with the actually achieved limitation of infarct size, contrast angiography 1 month after myocardial infarction revealed a relatively larger improvement in left ventricular function. There was a trend of benefit also in patients treated more than 3 hours after symptom onset.

Figure 13 shows the regional dyssynergic area of the left ventricle for streptokinase and placebo patients in relation to the size of the area at risk at baseline. There was a highly significant linear relationship between the sum of ST-segment elevation in the pre-randomization ECG and the extent of the regional wall motion abnormalities 1 month after myocardial infarction. A similar relationship was also present for the global ejection fraction, the enzyme and ECG-infarct size. In all subgroups the infarct size in streptokinase treated patients was smaller than in those who were not so treated. The magnitude of the sum of ST-segment elevations at baseline was also a strong prognosticator of short- and long-term mortality.[7]

Impact of late vessel patency in patients without early reperfusion

A peaking of MB-CK $\leq$ 15 hours or $>$ 15 hours after symptom onset differentiates patients with drug-induced or spontaneous early reperfusion from those without early reperfusion.[5,8–14] This

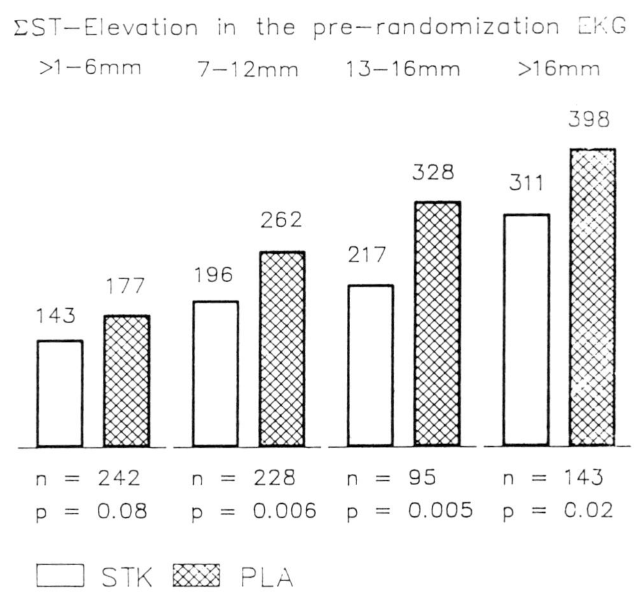

Figure 13 *Angio infarct size in relation to the area at risk*

Table 1 *Baseline characteristics of all patients with an MB-CK peak of > 15 h (average 21±4 h) after symptom onset. Comparison between patients in whom, at angiography 31±12 days after acute myocardial infarction, the infarct-related coronary artery was patent or occluded. Percentages of patients (in parentheses: actual numbers) or mean values ± SD of continuous variables are presented.*

Infarct-related coronary artery	*Patent*	*Occluded*	*p-value*
Number of patients	215	153	
Medical history			
Hypertension	18 (39)	21 (32)	n.s.
Previous MI	6 (13)	6 (9)	n.s.
Cardiac failure	17 (36)	15 (23)	n.s.
Diabetes mellitus	8 (17)	7 (10)	n.s.
Conditions at randomization			
Age (yr)	54.9 ± 9.8	54.8 ± 8.5	n.s.
Female	14 (29)	14 (21)	n.s.
Bundle branch block	2 (5)	3 (5)	n.s.
Site of infarction			
Anterior	38 (81)	37 (56)	
Inferior	61 (132)	63 (96)	
Undefined	1 (2)	1 (1)	n.s.
Heart rate (min.)	76.7±17.5	77.1±16.4	n.s.
Systol. blood pressure (mmHg)	137±29	138±26	n.s.
Diast. blood pressure (mmHg)	85±17	85±16	n.s.
Time symptom onset to treatment (min.)	185±76	186±76	n.s.
Ischemic area at risk (ΣST-elevation, mm)	11.2±8.5	9.8±7.9	n.s.
Actual developed infarct size			
MB-CK area (IU/L×h)	1835±1250	1780±998	n.s.
QRS-score	35.8±25	33.4±19	n.s.
Left ventricular function at 4 weeks			
Global EF (%)	56.1±13.4	49.8±13.8	0.000
Regional DA (square units)	239±182	324±192	0.000

report deals with a cohort of 368 patients of the ISAM study, in whom according to a late peaking in the serum time-activity curve spontaneous or drug-induced early reperfusion had not occurred. Patients who still had a patent infarct artery 1 month later may be considered comparable with patients reperfused late by delayed thrombolysis.

In Table 1 characteristics are listed for all patients in whom the serum MB-CK activity peaked more than 15 hours after onset of symptoms. The mean value of 21 ± 4 hours is in keeping with the findings in patients with angiographically proven persistent occlusion.[8–14] Comparison is made for patients in whom the infarct-related coronary artery was either patent or occluded at angiography 1 month later. There was no difference between patent and occluded artery groups

Figure 14 *Late MB-CK peaker*

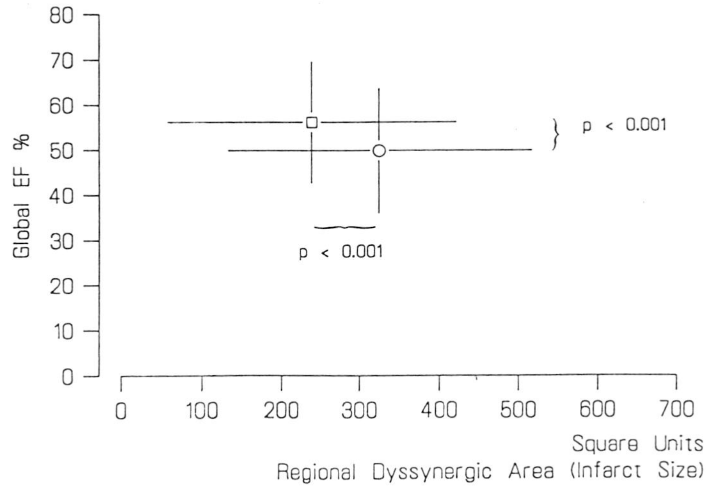

Left ventricular function 1 month after MI (all patients, n=368). Infarct-related artery: patent □, occluded ○

with regard to medical history or conditions at randomization. There was a trend both to a larger size of the ischemic area at baseline and also to larger acutely developed infarct sizes according to the MB-CK area or the QRS score respectively, in patients in whom the infarct-related artery was patent at 1 month.

Nevertheless at 1 month left ventricular function determined by global ejection fraction and regional dyssynergic area was improved to a highly significant degree in patients who had a patent infarct-related coronary artery as compared with those in whom the arteries were found to be still occluded.

In Table 2 patients treated with streptokinase and placebo are compared separately. Again, there was no significant difference in all baseline variables, but significant differences in left ventricular function 1 month later. Late 'spontaneous' reperfusion occurred in 74 of 116 (64%) streptokinase treated patients as compared with 141 of 252 (56%) patients without thrombolytic therapy. Patients who had an occluded infarct-related artery either treated with thrombolysis or not, had a somewhat larger size of the ischemic area at risk. Accordingly, in the placebo group the developed infarct sizes tended to be larger as compared with those in whom the vessel was occluded. In thrombolysed patients, however, the developed infarct sizes tended to be smaller in the patent coronary artery group. This finding is consistent with the suggestion that although late reperfusion had not occurred early enough to influence the MB-CK curve, thrombolytic therapy still might have limited somewhat the acutely developed infarct size.

Left ventricular function 1 month after myocardial infarction in late enzyme peakers

Figure 14 shows the comparison in global ejection fraction and regional dyssynergic area for the total group of patients 1 month after myocardial infarction in whom the infarct-related coronary artery was patent or occluded. Figure 15 shows the same for the subgroup of patients given streptokinase, Figure 16 for those without thrombolytic therapy, and Figure 17 for patients in whom the proximal left anterior descending coronary artery was affected. There were highly significant differences in patients in whom a late reperfusion of the infarct-related coronary artery had or had not occurred. The magnitude of these differences in all subgroups (although those are not shown here) was the same as in the total group. A patent infarct-related coronary artery was of

Table 2 *Characteristics of patients with an MB-CK peak of > 15 h in whom at angiography 1 month after acute myocardial infarction the infarct-related coronary artery was patent or occluded. Comparison between streptokinase (STK) treated or placebo (PLA) patients.*

	STK			*PLA*		
	Patent	*Occluded*	*p-value*	*Patent*	*Occluded*	*p-value*
Number of patients	74	42		141	111	
Site of infarction						
Anterior	32%(24)	21%(9)		40%(57)	42%(47)	
Inferior	65%(48)	79%(33)		60%(84)	57%(63)	
Undefined	3%(2)	0 (0)	n.s.	0(0)	1%(1)	n.s.
Time symptom onset to treatment (min.)	192 ± 82	185 ± 74	n.s.	182 ± 73	187 ± 77	n.s.
Ischemic area at risk (EST-elevation, mm)	9.9 ± 7.8	8.7 ± 5.6	n.s.	11.8 ± 8.8	10.3 ± 8.5	n.s.
Actual developed infarct size						
MB-CK area (IU/L × h)	$1463^{*} \pm 1063$	1680 ± 1040	n.s.	$2029^{*} \pm 1299$	1819 ± 984	n.s.
QRS-score	$30.9^{**} \pm 20$	32.1 ± 15	n.s.	$38.4^{**} \pm 27$	34.0 ± 20	n.s.
Left ventricular function at 4 weeks						
Global EF (%)	58.8 ± 12.8	53.0 ± 13.6	<0.03	54.7 ± 13.5	48.6 ± 13.8	0.001
Regional DA (square units)	204 ± 165	273 ± 155	<0.03	258 ± 188	344 ± 201	0.001

* $p < 0.001$, ** $p < 0.03$ patent STK versus patent PLA

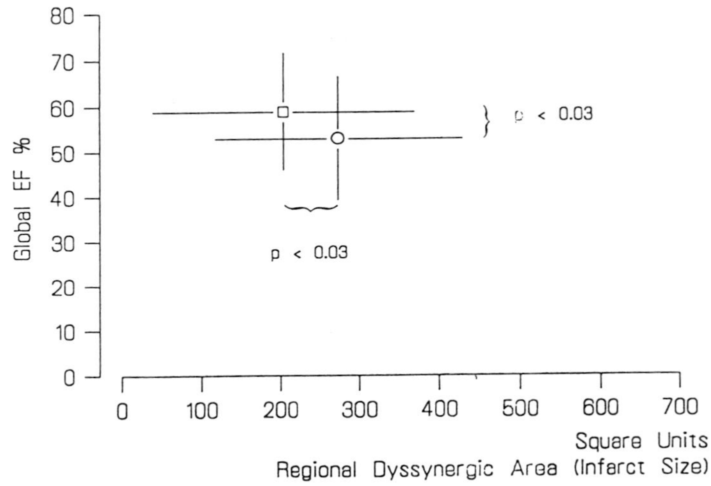

Figure 15 *Late MB-CK peaker: left ventricular function 1 month after MI (STK-Group, n=116). Infarct related artery: patent □, occluded ○*

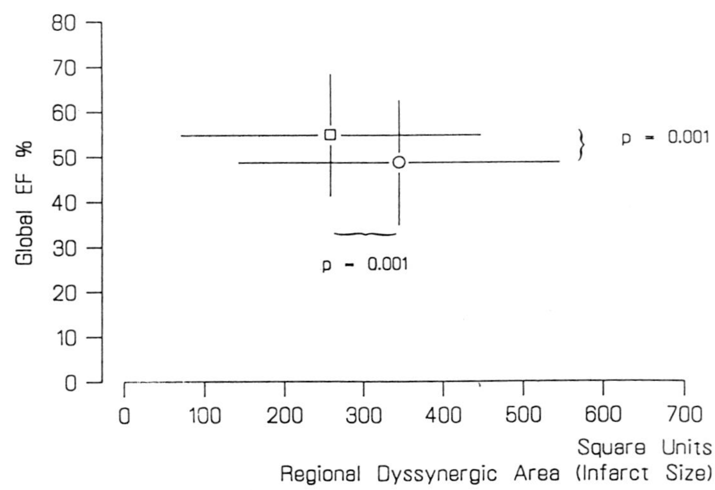

Figure 16 *Late MB-CK peaker: left ventricular function 1 month after MI (PLA-group, n=253). Infarct-related artery: patent □, occluded ○*

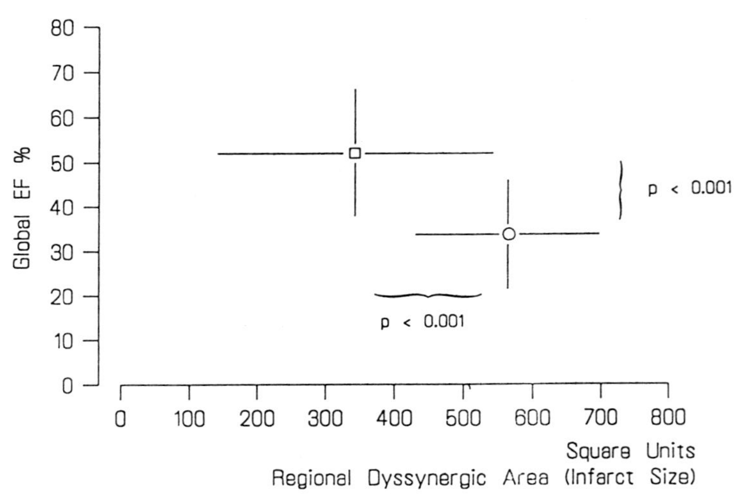

Figure 17 *Late MB-CK peaker: left ventricular function 1 month after MI (Prox-LAD, n=64). Infarct-relaxed artery: patent □, occluded ○*

benefit regardless of whether patients had been treated with streptokinase or not, and whether the infarct-related vessel was the left anterior descending, the circumflex, or the right coronary artery. Since there were no differences between all other variables tested (Tables 1 and 2), the better left ventricular function 1 month after acute myocardial infarction can only be caused by one factor, that is patency of the infarct-related coronary artery.

Discussion

The major predictor of long-term survival after myocardial infarction is the status of left ventricular function at hospital discharge. Actual salvage of ischemic myocardium and limitation of infarct size is predominantly the result of timely reperfusion. If treatment was initiated within 3–4 hours after the onset of symptoms of myocardial infarction, limitation of the infarct size had been demonstrated with various thrombolytic agents. The results shown here are consistent with this. If initiation of thrombolytic therapy was delayed for more than 4 hours, salvage was modest or not discernible at all.[5, 7, 15–18] The mechanisms by which thrombolysis improves survival in patients with myocardial infarction up to 24 hours' duration[19] are not fully understood.

The syndrome of 'hibernating' myocardium

The highly beneficial effect of late perfusion to the zone of infarcted myocardium, as shown in this chapter, might best be explained by the syndrome of hibernating myocardium.[20] Particularly in regions bordering the zone of irreversible necrosis[21] there may be myocardial perfusion which is chronically reduced but still sufficient to maintain viability of the tissue. Myocardial function may remain impaired permanently or for as long as myocardial perfusion is inadequate.[20]

Other observations which fit this hypothesis include the finding that those patients who after thrombolytic therapy achieved completely adequate reperfusion by early coronary artery bypass grafting had a greater long-term survival and better left ventricular function than comparable patients who did not undergo surgery.[22–24] Similarly, long-term follow-up of patients after successful PTCA of a high-grade residual infarct artery stenosis performed some days[25, 26] or even months after an acute myocardial infarction treated with or without thrombolysis[26, 27] showed significant improvement of left ventricular function.

Clinical implications

Early reperfusion is critical for achieving maximal salvage of jeopardized myocardium ('direct limitation of infarct size'). Our data strongly suggest that late reperfusion of an infarct-related artery has a potential additive impact on preservation of left ventricular function either by improvement of function, prevention of subsequent deterioration, or both ('indirect limitation of infarct size').

Left ventricular function at hospital discharge is the most powerful predictor of long-term survival. The large differences in global and regional ejection fraction 1 month after infarction between patients with a non-perfused artery and an artery that was perfused during the healing phase of an acute myocardial infarction underscore the importance of restoration of an adequate flow even too late to prevent acute myocardial damage.

The potential of reversible left ventricular dysfunction late after acute myocardial infarction may suggest a more aggressive revascularization approach in patients with persistent infarct artery occlusion. However, the risk/benefit ratio should be carefully weighed for each individual patient.

References

1. ISIS-2 (Second International Study of Infarct Survival) Collaborative Group. Randomised trial of intravenous streptokinase, oral aspirin, both, or neither among 17,187 cases of suspected acute myocardial infarction: ISIS-2. *Lancet i*, 1988, 349–360.
2. Stadius M L, Davis K, Maynard C, Ritchie J L, Kennedy J W, Risk stratification for 1 year survival based on characteristics identified in the early hours of acute myocardial infarction. *Circulation 4*, 1986, 703–711.
3. Dalen J E, Gore J M, Braunwald E, Borer J, Goldberg R J, Passamani E R, Forman S, Knatterud G, and the TIMI investigators. Six- and twelve-month follow-up of the Phase I Thrombolysis in Myocardial Infarction (TIMI) Trial. *Am. J. Cardiol. 62*, 1988, 179–185.
4. Betriu A, Castaner A, Sanz G A, Pare J C, Roig E, Coll S, Magrina J, Navarro-Lopez F, Angiographic findings 1 month after myocardial infarction: A prospective study of 259 survivors. *Circulation 65*, 1982, 1099–1105.
5. The I.S.A.M. Study Group. A prospective trial of intravenous streptokinase in acute myocardial infarction (I.S.A.M.). Mortality, morbidity, and infarct size at 21 days. *N. Engl. J. Med. 314*, 1986, 1465–1471.
6. Schröder R, Neuhaus K L, Leizorovicz A, Linderer T, Tebbe U, for the ISAM Study Group. A prospective placebo-controlled double-blind multicenter trial of intravenous streptokinase in acute myocardial infarction (ISAM): Long-term mortality and morbidity. *JACC 9*, 1987, 197–203.
7. Schröder R, Neuhaus K L, Linderer T, Tebbe U, Brüggemann T, Wegscheider K, Thrombolysis-induced limitation of infarct size in relation to time from pain onset and infarct localization: Results from the ISAM Study. *JACC 13(2)*, 1989, 95A (abstr).
8. Ganz W, Geft I, Maddahi J, Berman D, Charuzi Y, Shah P K, Swan H J, Norsurgical reperfusion in evolving myocardial infarction. *JACC 1(5)*, 1983, 1247–1253.
9. Ong L, Reiser P, Coromilas J, Scherr L, Morrison J, Left ventricular function and rapid release of creatine kinase MB in acute myocardial infarction. *N. Engl. J. Med. 309*, 1983, 1–6.
10. Schröder R, Biamino G, von Leitner E R, Linderer T, Brüggemann T, Heitz J, Vöhringer H F, Wegscheider K, Intravenous short-term infusion of streptokinase in acute myocardial infarction. *Circulation 67*, 1983, 536–548.
11. Gore J M, Roberts R, Ball S P, Montero A, Goldberg R J, Dalen J E, Peak creatine kinase as a measure of effectiveness of thrombolytic therapy in acute myocardial infarction. *Am. J. Cardiol. 59*, 1987, 1234–1238.
12. Lewis B S, Ganz W, Laramee P, Cercek B, Hod H, Shah P K, Lew A S, Usefulness of a rapid initial increase in plasma creatine kinase activity as a marker of reperfusion during thrombolytic therapy for acute myocardial infarction. *Am. J. Cardiol. 62*, 1988, 20–24.
13. Garabedian H D, Gold H K, Yasuda T, Johns J, Finkelstein D M, Gaivin R J, Cobbaert C, Leinbach R C, Collen D, Detection of coronary artery reperfusion with creatine kinase-MB determinations during thrombolytic therapy: Correlation with acute angiography. *JACC 11*, 1988, 729–739.
14. Hirai T, Fujita M, Sasayama S, Ohno A, Yamanishi H, Asanoi H, Importance of coronary collateral circulation for kinetics of serum creatine kinase in acute myocardial infarction. *Am. J. Cardiol. 60*, 1987, 446–450.
15. Verani A S, Roberts R, Preservation of cardiac function by coronary thrombolysis during acute myocardial infarction: Fact or myth? *JACC 10*, 1987, 470–476.

16. Patel B, Kloner R A, Analysis of reported randomized trials of streptokinase for acute myocardial infarction in the 1980s. *Am. J. Cardiol. 59*, 1987, 501–504.
17. Chesebro J H, Knatterud G, Roberts R, Borer J, Cohen L S, Dalen J, Dodge H T, Francis C K, Hills D, Ludbrook P, Markis J E, Mueller H, Passamani E, Powers E R, Rao A K, Robertson T, Ross A, Ryan T J, Sobel B E, Willerson J, Williams D O, Zaret B L, Braunwald E, Thrombolysis in myocardial infarction (TIMI) trial, phase I: A comparison between intravenous tissue plasminogen activator and intravenous streptokinase. Clinical findings through hospital discharge. *Circulation 76*, 1987, 142–154.
18. Sheehan F H, Mathey D G, Schofer J, Dodge H T, Bolson E L, Factors that determine recovery of left ventricular function after thrombolysis in patients with acute myocardial infarction. *Circulation 71*, 1985, 1121–1128.
19. The Multicenter Postinfarction Research Group. Risk stratification and survival after myocardial infarction. *N. Engl. J. Med. 309*, 1983, 331–336.
20. Braunwald E, Rutherford J D, Reversible ischemic left ventricular dysfunction: Evidence for the 'hibernating myocardium'. *JACC 6*, 1986, 1467–1470.
21. Sheehan F H, Doerr R, Schmidt W G, Bolson E L, Uebis R, von Essen R, Effert S, Dodge H T, Early recovery of left ventricular function after thrombolytic therapy for acute myocardial infarction: An important determinant of survival. *JACC 12*, 1988, 289–300.
22. Sutton J M, Taylor G J, Mikell F L, Moses H W, Korsmeyer C, Dove J T, Batchelder J E, Wellons Jr. H A, Schneider J A, Thrombolytic therapy followed by early revascularization for acute myocardial infarction. *Am. J. Cardiol. 57*, 1986, 1227–1231.
23. Mathey D G, Schofer J, Sheehan F H, Krebber H J, Justen M, Rodewald G, Dodge H T, Bleifeld W, Improved survival up to four years after early coronary thrombolysis *Am. J. Cardiol. 61*, 1988, 524–529.
24. Kereiakes D J, Topol E J, George B S, Abbottsmith C W, Stack R S, Candela R J, O'Neill W W, Martin L H, Califf R M, and the TAMI Study Group. Emergency coronary artery bypass surgery preserves global and regional left ventricular function after intravenous tissue plasminogen activator therapy for acute myocardial infarction. *JACC 11*, 1988, 899–907.
25. Guerci A D, Gerstenblith G, Brinker J A, Chandra N C, Gottlieb S O, Bahr R D, Weiss J L, Shapiro E P, Flaherty J T, Bush E D, Chew P H, Gottlieb S H, Halperien H R, Ouyang P, Walford G D, Bell W R, Fatterpacker A K, Liewellyn A, Topol E J, Healy B, Siu C, Becker L C, Weisfeld M L, A randomized trial of intravenous tissue plasminogen activator for acute myocardial infarction with subsequent randomization to elective coronary angioplasty. *N. Engl. J. Med. 317*, 1987, 1613–1618.
26. Guhl B, Schnitzer L, Brüggemann T, Linderer T, Spielberg C, Schröder R, Left-ventricular function 6 months after PTCA performed early or late after acute myocardial infarction and in patients without myocardial infarction. *Eur. Heart. J. 9* (Supplement 1) 1988, 104 (abstr.).
27. Rosenheck S, Hasin Y, Masseri M, Improvement in left ventricular function following percutaneous transluminal angioplasty performed several months post transmural myocardial infarction treated with streptokinase. *Circulation 74*-II, 1986, 123 (abstr.).

Chapter 5

THE CLINICAL DEVELOPMENT OF RECOMBINANT TISSUE PLASMINOGEN ACTIVATOR (rt-PA, ALTEPLASE)

Elliott B. Grossbard and Alan Hopkins

Genentech, Inc, San Francisco, CA, USA

Introduction

In March of 1983 the first published description of the cloning and expression of recombinant tissue plasminogen activator (rt-PA) appeared in *Nature*;[1] less than 1 year later the first clinical trial with rt-PA was initiated. Over the ensuing four years, thousands of patients were treated with rt-PA in trials that established its utility in inducing coronary thrombolysis,[2,3] reducing infarct size,[4] preserving ventricular function[4–7], and reducing mortality[8] in patients suffering an acute myocardial infarction. Since the results of these trials are well described in this volume and elsewhere, this review will focus on some insights provided by the Genentech data base, as well as update studies with rt-PA (alteplase, Activase ®, Actilyse) in indications other than acute myocardial infarction.

Table 1 *Baseline characteristics of rt-PA patients*

Variable	*No.*[1]	
Age (years)	1180	
Mean±S.D.[2]		55.4±10.2
Range		23–75
Weight(kg)	919	
Mean±S.D.		80.9±15.3
Range		42–155
Gender		
Male	936	79.3%
Female	244	20.7%
Infarct Artery		
CIR[3]	128	10.8%
LAD[4]	518	43.9%
RCA[5]	507	43.0%
Normal	11	0.9%
Unknown	16	1.4%
Interval from pain to treatment (hr)		
±S.D.	1172	3.8±1.5

1 numbers vary due to absent data points
2 standard deviation
3 left circumflex artery
4 left anterior descending artery
5 right coronary artery

The data base covers some 1,500 patients from studies that have for the most part been independently reported.[2–5, 9–11]

Studies in myocardial infarction

Coronary thrombolysis

The demographics of the pooled group of patients are displayed in Table 1 and are characteristic of the kinds of patients generally studied in coronary thrombolysis trials: a mean age of 55, approximately 80 kilograms in weight, predominantly male, location of the infarct artery evenly divided between the territories of the left anterior descending and right coronary arteries, and an interval from pain onset to treatment of slightly less than 4 hours.

Table 2 *30 day mortality by IRA[1] patency*

Patency	*Death* No(%)	Yes(%)
No	242(91)	24(9)
Yes	643(96)	26(4)

[1] Infarct related artery–patency at 90 minute angiogram. $P<.001$

A retrospective review of our data base demonstrated a very strong association between infarct artery patency 90 minutes following treatment and in-hospital survival (Table 2), an observation made by others in smaller individual trials.[11,12] We therefore reviewed some factors that might alter efficacy with regard to coronary thrombolysis. The rt-PA used in the early trials was produced in roller bottles (RB rt-PA) and was predominantly two-chain in composition. Several investigators noted that the predominantly single chain rt-PA, produced in large scale suspension culture (SC rt-PA), introduced in 1985 had a more rapid clearance from the circulation and thus required a higher dose for equivalent efficacy.[3,13] We found, after allowing for the pharmacokinetic difference, that both types of rt-PA were effective as long as the therapeutic dose for the respective type was administered, i.e., at least 50 mg of RB rt-PA and at least 70 mg of SC rt-PA over the first 90 minutes (Table 3).

Table 3 *Efficacy analysis: RB[1] versus SC[2] rt-PA*

	Number Occluded[3](%)	*Number Patent[3](%)*
RB rt-PA	103 (32)	217 (68)
SC rt-PA	186 (28)	483 (72)
TOTAL	289 (29)	700 (71)

[1] at least 50 mg over 90 minutes
[2] at least 70 mg over 90 minutes
[3] at 90 minute angiogram

RB rt-PA = rt-PA produced in roller bottles
SC rt-PA = rt-PA produced in large scale suspension culture

We next looked at the relationship between time to treatment and thrombolytic efficacy. Others had observed an inverse relationship, both for streptokinase and anistreplase, between time to treatment and coronary thrombolytic efficacy.[2,14] With rt-PA we found that although there was a slight trend to greater efficacy in the first two hours, there was no significant diminution of efficacy up to 6–9 hours (Table 4).

Table 4 *Efficacy of rt-PA: patency[1] time to treatment*

Time (hr)	*No.*	*Occluded(%)*	*Patent[1] (%)*
0–1	11	18	82
1–2	98	20	80
2–3	258	28	72
3–4	245	29	71
4–5	129	31	69
5–6	79	18	82
6–9	41	29	71

1. 90 minute angiogram

Since most trials in which rt-PA was studied involved fixed dosing (i.e. not on mg/kg body weight basis), we sought to discover in retrospect whether those patients who had received a higher weight-adjusted dose had demonstrated a higher incidence of infarct artery patency following treatment. Consistent with reports in the literature,[15] it does seem possible to increase the coronary thrombolytic efficacy of rt-PA by increasing the dose per kilogram body weight over the first 90 minutes. Recent data from Germany[16] suggest that a dose of 100 mg over 90 minutes is associated with a patency rate of 90% at 90 minutes (without a high reocclusion rate) which also supports this concept (Table 5).

Table 5 *Efficacy of rt-PA: patency[1] dose by weight*

Dose (mg/kg)	*No.*	*Patent[1] (%)*
<0.8	134	55
0.8–1.0	357	70
1.0–1.2	258	78
>1.2	110	83

1. 90 minute angiogram

Bleeding

It is far more difficult to pool data on bleeding events than on coronary thrombolysis, because the interpretation of an event as serious or severe is much more subjective, less amenable to central analysis, and less uniform between studies. Consequently, the data presented here should be used for the purpose of hypothesis development, rather than as a basis for firm conclusions. It has been reported that a dose of rt-PA of 150 mg over 6 hours is associated with an incidence of intracerebral bleeding in the range of 1.5–2%,[17,18] more than threefold that observed with the dose of 100 mg over 3–6 hours. When we include patients treated with up to 150 mg of rt-PA in our review, there is a strong suggestion of increased risk of major bleeding as patients get older, particularly for those over 70. This trend is not apparent when only patients treated with 100 mg are included (Table 6). Not surprisingly, there is a trend to increased bleeding when the dose exceeds 1.25 mg/kg, and when the patients are female (Table 6). Because these data are derived from populations treated with fixed doses (and include patients treated with 150 mg of rt-PA) and because females tend to weigh less, it is likely that an interaction between these variables accounts at least in part for the increased bleeding seen in females. The majority of these bleeds were from catheterization sites, and thus unlikely to be a problem in routine clinial practice.

Table 6 *Bleeding: age, gender, dose*

	All Patients		*100 mg*	
Age	*No.*	*'Major' bleeds (%)*	*No.*	*'Major' bleeds (%)*
35–45	293	3.8	107	7.5
46–55	473	3.6	197	4.1
56–65	589	6.6	302	7.3
66–70	206	8.3	98	8.2
71–75	114	13.2	41	7.3
Gender				
Male	1393	5.1		
Female	304	9.2		
Dose (mg/kg)				
≤1.25	423	4.7		
>1.25	1254	6.3		

In summary, the data base suggests that a strong correlation exists between infarct artery patency and in-hospital survival, that rt-PA maintains its coronary thrombolytic efficacy for many hours after the onset of chest pain, that increasing the dose in the first 90 minutes improves the patency rate, but that increasing the total dose increases serious bleeding as well. There is no unequivocal data that bleeding incidence is related to age or gender. Furthermore, heparin that was administered along with rt-PA in these studies must certainly contribute to the bleeding that is observed during thrombolytic therapy. Its role as adjunctive therapy remains to be established definitively.

Studies in Other Indications

Pulmonary Embolism

Thrombolytic therapy was initially approved by the US Food and Drug Administration for use in pulmonary embolism. Though widespread clinical acceptance did not follow, considerable interest still exists in the use of rt-PA in this condition. Three studies have been published to date.[19–21] Utilizing pulmonary angiography as the principal method of patient selection and evaluation, the three studies reached the following tentative conclusions: a) that a dose of rt-PA of 50–100 mg over 2–7 hours was capable of producing significant angiographic and hemodynamic improvement; b) that the intravenous route of infusion was as effective as the intrapulmonary; and c) that rt-PA was significantly more effective than the standard dose of urokinase (Table 7).

At present four more studies are under way or near completion. One, at McMaster University in Canada, is studying a bolus dose of rt-PA (0.6 mg/kg over 1–2 minutes) compared with placebo, using lung scans at 24 hours to evaluate outcome. One is using angiography to compare rt-PA with a high dose short infusion of urokinase. The third is comparing rt-PA with heparin for effects on right ventricular function and wall motion as assessed by echocardiography. The fourth is comparing rt-PA with the standard dose of urokinase for effects on pulmonary hemodynamics. The results of these trials should increase significantly our understanding of the utility of rt-PA in acute pulmonary embolism.

Table 7 *Studies in pulmonary embolism*

Investigator	*Dose (mg)*	*Duration (hr)*	*No.*	*Control*	*Endpoint*
Goldhaber (19b)	50–90	2–6	47	–	angiography
Verstraete (20)	50–100	2–7	34	IV[1]/IPA[1]	angiography
Goldhaber (21)	100	2	45	UK	angiography

[1] IV = intravenous; IPA = intrapulmonary artery

Unstable Angina

We have substantial evidence that thrombus is involved in the clinical syndrome of unstable angina. Since this syndrome has a high rate of progression to acute myocardial infarction, great enthusiasm has been shown for the study of thrombolytic therapy in unstable angina. Several trials have been published on the effects of rt-PA in unstable angina.[22–26] Though there are some contradictory results, some tentative conclusions can be drawn: a) that in patients without a visible thrombus there is little angiographic improvement attributable to rt-PA that would not occur naturally or with heparin treatment; b) that some patients with significant thrombi can have dramatic responses with appreciable angiographic improvement and clinical stabilization, superior to that observed with heparin, obviating the need for angioplasty or surgery;[27] c) that certain patients refractory to heparin and aspirin may be stabilized by rt-PA; and d) that it will take very large clinical trials to establish the role, if any, of rt-PA in unstable angina (Table 8).

Table 8 *Studies in unstable angina*

Investigator	*Dose*	*Duration (hr)*	*No.*	*Control*	*Endpoint*
Gold (22)	1.75mg/kg	12	24	placebo	angiography
Nicklas (23)	1.50 mg	8	40	placebo	pacing threshold
Ardissino (24)	100 mg	3	24	placebo	clinical
Topol (26)	60, 100 mg	1, 6	66	placebo	angiography
de Zwaan (25)	100 mg	3	20	—	angiography

Such a trial, the TIMI-3 trial, is planned and is expected to begin this fall. It will seek to ascertain the role of rt-PA and angioplasty in the treatment of unstable angina, assuming that heparin and aspirin are administered to all patients.

Deep Vein Thrombosis

Several small studies have been concluded utilizing rt-PA in the treatment of deep vein thrombosis of the legs.[28,30] The doses have varied from approximately 40 mg up to 150 mg, and the durations have ranged from 4 to 24 hours; the infusions have been continuous or interrupted. It is difficult to draw any conclusions from such fragmentary data. Nevertheless, it appears that: a) continuous infusions of a low dose of rt-PA are not clearly superior to a shorter infusion of the same or even a lower total dose; b) an optimal dose and duration of therapy has not been identified; c) the relationship between successful thrombolysis and the reduction in the incidence and in the morbidity of the post-phlebitic syndrome needs to be established more definitively (Table 9).

Table 9 *Studies in deep vein thrombosis*

Investigator	*Dose*	*Duration (hr)*	*No.*	*Control*	*Endpoint*
Turpie (28)	0.5 mg/kg	4	24	placebo/heparin	venography
Turpie (28)	0.5 mg/kg×2	8	53	placebo/heparin	venography
Goldhaber (30)	1.2 mg/kg	24	65	heparin	venography
Verhaeghe (29)	100–150	8×2	32	placebo	venography

Peripheral Artery Occlusion

Studies with rt-PA in peripheral artery occlusion are few.[31–33] These studies all indicate that a high degree of thrombolysis can be achieved with local infusion of a relatively small dose of rt-PA via an infusion catheter placed within or adjacent to an angiographically visualized thrombus. Whether this form of therapy is preferable to, adjunctive to, or merely an alternative to surgery in selected cases has not been established (Table 10).

Table 10 *Studies in peripheral arterial occlusion*

Investigator	*Dose*	*Duration (hr)*	*No.*	*Control*	*Endpoint*
Graor (31)	0.05 mg/kg/hr	4–8	65	–	angiography
Verstraete (32)	10 mg/hr	up to 5	50	–	angiography
Goldhaber (33)	10 mg/bolus 5/mg/hr	up to 24	22	UK	angiography

Thromboembolic Stroke

A major pilot study is under way in the U.S. assessing the feasibility of a trial of rt-PA in acute thromboembolic stroke. More than 75 patients have been enrolled to date with encouraging responses in 30–35% of patients. Perhaps as important is the very low morbidity observed in this trial with the use of rt-PA. A very low rate (under 5%) of evolution to haemorrhagic stroke has been observed. A placebo controlled trial is planned for the fall of 1989 or early 1990.

Retinal Vein Occlusion

An open pilot study of over 50 patients at Johns Hopkins Hospital and the University of Maryland has concluded that there may be long-term improvement of visual acuity following treatment of patients with retinal vein occlusion with rt-PA.[34] This observation needs to be confirmed in properly controlled trials.

Conclusion

Much has been learned over the past five years about the use of rt-PA in myocardial infarction. Appreciable benefits have been described in terms of survival and heart function. The coming years will see additions to this fund of knowledge, and, it is hoped, fresh benefits to patients with other indications for treatment.

References

1. Pennica D, Holmes W E, Harkins R N, Vehar G A, Ward C A, Bennett W F, Yelverton E, Seeburg P H, Heyneker H L, Goeddel D V, Collen D, Cloning and expression of human tissue-type plasminogen activator cDNA in E. Coli. *Nature 301*, 1983, 214–221.
2. Chesebro J H, Knatterud G, Roberts R, Borer J, Cohen L S, Dalen J, Dodge H T, Francis C K, Hillis D, Ludbrook P A, Markis J E, Mueller H, Passamani E R, Powers E R, Rao A K, Robertson T, Ryan T J, Ross A, Sobel B E, Willerson J T, Williams D O, Zaret B L, Braunwald E, Thrombolysis in myocardial infarction (TIMI) trial, phase l: a comparison between intravenous tissue plasminogen activator and intravenous strepkotinase. *Circulation 76*, 1987, 142–154.
3. Mueller H S, Rao A K, Forman S A, Comparative studies of coronary reperfusion and systemic fibrinogenolysis with two forms of recombinant tissue plasminogen activator. *J Am Coll Cardiol 10*, 1987, 479–490.
4. Van de Werf F, Arnold A E R, and the European Cooperative Study Group for recombinant tissue plasminogen activator. Intravenous tissue plasminogen activator and size of infarct, left ventricular function, and survival in acute myocardial infarction. *Br Med J 297*, 1988, 1374–1379.
5. Guerci A D, Gerstenblith G, Brinker J A, Chandra N C, Gottlieb S O, Bahr R D, Weis J L, Shapiro E T, Flaherty J T, Bush D E, Chew P H, Gottlieb S H, Halperin H R, Ouyang P, Walford G D, Bell W R, Flatterpaker A K, Llewellyn M, Topol E J, Healy B, Siu C O, Becker L C, Weisfeldt M L, A randomized trial of intravenous tissue plasminogen activator for acute myocardial infarction with subsequent randomization to elective coronary angioplasty. *New Engl J Med 317*, 1987, 1613–1618.
6. O'Rourke M, Baron D, Keogh A, Kelly R, Nelson G, Barnes C, Raftos J, Graham K, Hillman K, Newman H, Healey J, Wooridge J, White H, Whitlock R, Norris R, Limitation of myocardial infarction by early infusion of recombinant tissue-type plasminogen activator. *Circulation 77*, 1988, 1311–1315.
7. National Heart Foundation of Australia Coronary Thrombolysis Group. Coronary thrombolysis and myocardial salvage by tissue plasminogen activator given up to four hours after onset of myocardial infarction. *Lancet i*, 1988, 203–207.

8. Wilcox R G, Von der Liffe G, Olsson C G, Jensen G, Skene A M, Hampton J R, Trial of tissue plasminogen activator for mortality reduction in acute myocardial infarction. Anglo-Scandinavian Study of Early Thrombolysis (ASSET). *Lancet ii*, 1988, 525–530.
9. Topol E J, Morris D C, Smalling R W, Schumacher R R, Taylor C R, Nishikawa A, Liberman H, Collen D C, Tufte M E, Grossbard E, O'Neill W W, A multicenter randomized placebo-controlled trial of a new form of intravenous recombinant tissue-type plasminogen activator (Activase®) in acute myocardial infarction. *J Am Coll Cardiol 9*, 1987, 1205–1213.
10. Passamani E, Hodges M, Herman M, Grose R, Chaitman B, Rogers W, Forman S, Terrin M, Knatterud G, Robertson T, Braunwald E, The thrombolysis in myocardial infarction (TIMI) phase II pilot study: tissue plasminogen activator followed by percutaneous transluminal coronary angioplasty. *J Am Coll Cardiol 10(5)*, 1987, 51B–64B.
11. Topol E J, Califf R M, George B S, Kereiakes D J, Abbottsmith C W, Candela R J, Lee K L, Pitt B, Stack R S, O'Neill W W, A multicenter randomized trial of intravenous tissue plasminogen activator and immediate angioplasty in acute myocardial infarction. *New Engl J Med 317*, 1987, 581–588.
12. Dalen J E, Gore J, Braunwald E, Borer J, Goldberg R J, Passamani E R, Forman S, Knatterud G, Six- and twelve-month follow-up of the thrombolysis in myocardial infarction (TIMI) trial. *Am J Cardiol 62*, 1988,179–185.
13. Garabedian H D, Gold H K, Leinbach R C, Johns J A, Yasuda T, Kanke M, Collen D C, Comparative properties of two preparations of recombinant tissue-type plasminogen activator in patients with acute myocardial infarction. *J Am Cardiol 9*, 1987, 599–607.
14. Anderson J L, Rothbard R L, Hackworthy R A, Sorensen S G, Fitzpatrick P G, Dahl C F, Hagan A D, Browne K F, Synkoviak G P, Menlove R L, Barry W H, Eckserson H W, Marder V J, Multicenter reperfusion trial of intravenous anisoylated plasminogen streptokinase activator complex (APSAC) in acute myocardial infarction: Controlled with comparison with intracoronary streptokinase. *J Am Coll Cardiol 11*, 1988, 1153–1163.
15. Topol E J, George B S, Kereiakes D J, Candela R J, Abbottsmith C W, Stump D S, Boswick J M, Stack R S, Califf R M, Comparison of two dose regimens of intravenous tissue plasminogen activator for acute myocardial infarction. *Am J Cardiol 61*, 1988, 723–728.
16. Neuhaus K L, Feuerer W, Jeep-Tebbe S, Niederer W, Vogt A, Tebbe U, Improved thrombolysis with rt-PA in acute myocardial infarction. *J Am Coll Cardiol 14*, 1989, 1566–1569.
17. Braunwald E, Knatterud G, Passamani E R, Robertson T, Solomon R, Update from the thrombolysis in myocardial infarction trial. *J Am Coll Cardiol 10*, 1987, 1970.
18. The TIMI Study Group. Comparison of invasive and conservative strategies after treatment with intravenous tissue plasminogen activator in acute myocardial infarction. *New Engl J Med 320*, 1989, 618–627.
19a. Goldhaber S Z, Vaughn D E, Markis J E, Selwyn A P, Meyerovitz M F, Loscalzo J, Kim D S, Kessler C M, Dawley D L, Sharma G V R K, Sasahara A, Grossbard E B, Braunwald E, Acute pulmonary embolism treated with tissue plasminogen activator. *Lancet ii*, 1986, 886–889.
19b. Goldhaber S Z, Meyerovitz M F, Markis J E, Kim D S, Kessler C M, Sharma G V R K, Vaughn D E, Selwyn A P, Dawley D L, Loscalzo J, Sashara A, Grossbard E B, Braunwald E, Thrombolytic therapy of acute pulmonary embolism: current status and future potential. *J Am Coll Cardiol 10(5)*, 10, 1987, 96B–104B.
20. Verstraete M, Miller G A H, Bounameaux H, Charbonnier B, Colle J P, Lecorf G, Marbet G A, Mombaerts P, Olsson C G, Intravenous and intrapulmonary recombinant tissue-type plasminogen activator in the treatment of acute massive pulmonary embolism. *Circulation 77*, 1988, 353–360.

21. Goldhaber S Z, Kessler C M, Heit J, Markis J, Sharma G V R K, Dawley D, Nagel J S, Meyerovitz M, Kim D, Vaughn D E, Parker J A, Tumeh S S, Drum D, Loscalzo J, Reagan K, Selwyn A P, Anderson J, Braunwald E, Randomized controlled trial of recombinant tissue plasminogen activator versus urokinase in the treatment of acute pulmonary embolism. *Lancet ii*, 1988, 293–298.
22. Gold H K, Johns J A, Leinbach R C, Yasuda T, Grossbard E, Zusman R, Collen D C, A randomized blinded placebo-controlled trial of recombinant human tissue-type plasminogen activator in patients with unstable angina pectoris. *Circulation 75*, 1987, 1192–1199.
23. Nicklas J M, Topol E J, Kander N, O'Neill W W, Walton J, Ellis S G, Gorman L, Pitt B, Randomized double-blind placebo-controlled trial of tissue plasminogen activator in unstable angina. *J Am Coll Cardiol 13*, 1989, 434–441.
24. Ardissino D, Specchia G, Barberis P, De Sevi S, Mussini A, Demicheli G, Montemartini C, Effect of rt-PA in unstable angina refractory to medical therapy. *Circulation 78(4)*, 1988, II–420.
25. de Zwaan C, Bar F W, Janssen J H A, de Swart H B, Vermeer F, Wellens H J J, Effect of thrombolytic therapy in unstable angina. *J Am Coll Cardiol 12*, 1988, 301–309.
26. Topol E J, Kleiman N S, Joelson Ellis S G, Wahl T, Califf R M, O'Brien M, Hopkins A, Roberts R, Williams D O, Tissue plasminogen activator for unstable angina pectoris: A multicenter randomized double-blind placebo-controlled trial. *J Am Coll Cardiol 13(2)*, 1989, 190A.
27. Topol E J, Nicklas J M, Kander N H, Walton J A, Ellis S G, Gorman L, Pitt B, Coronary revascularization after tissue plasminogen activator for unstable angina pectoris: results of a randomized double-blind placebo-controlled trial. *Am J Cardiol 62*, 1988, 368–371.
28. Turpie A G G, Thrombolysis in deep vein thrombosis. In *Thrombolysis in Cardiovascular Disease*, Julian D, Kubler W, Norris R M, Swan H J C, Collen D, Verstraete M (eds), Marcel Dekker Inc., New York, 1989, pp. 397–409.
29. Verhaeghe R, Besse P, Baunameaux H, Marbet G A, Multicenter pilot study of the efficacy and safety of systemic rt-PA administration in the treatment of deep vein thrombosis of the lower extremities and/or pelvis. *Thrombosis Research* (in press).
30. Goldhaber S Z, Meyerovitz M F, Green G, Citrin P, Heit J, Sobel M, Wheeler H B, Plante D, Kim H, Stump D, Hopkins A, Tufte M E, Braunwald E, A randomized controlled trial of tissue plasminogen activator in proximal deep vein thrombosis. *Am J Med* (in the press).
31. Graor R A, Olin J W, Regional thrombolysis in peripheral arterial occlusion. In *Thrombolysis in Cardiovascular Disease*, Julian D, Kubler W, Norris R M, Swan H J C, Collen D, Verstraete M (eds), Marcel Dekker Inc., New York, 1989, pp. 381–397.
32. Verstraete M, Hess H, Mahler F, Mietaschk A, Roth F J, Schneider E, Baert A L, Verhaege R. Femoro-popliteal artery thrombolysis with intra-arterial infusion of recombinant tissue-type plasminogen activator – report of a pilot trial. *Eur J Vasc Surg 2*, 1988, 155–159.
33. Goldhaber S Z, Meyerovitz M, Reagan K, Polak J, Kandarpa K, Grassi C, Bettmann M A, Whittemore A, Mannick J, Donaldson C M, Harrington D P, TPA versus urokinase: a randomized controlled trial in peripheral arterial occlusion. *Circulation 78(4)*, 1988, II-270.
34. Elman M J, Quinlan P M, Fine S L, Shapiro E, Weisfeldt M, Enger C, Thrombolytic Therapy for Central Retinal Vein Occlusion. Submitted for publication.

Chapter 6

THE BALANCE BETWEEN RISK AND BENEFIT WITH rt-PA – INCLUDING WELLCOME'S EXPERIENCE IN TRIALS IN ACUTE MYOCARDIAL INFARCTION

Alasdair D. Malcolm

Wellcome Research Laboratories, Beckenham, UK

Introduction

The experience now accumulated in clinical trials with recombinant tissue plasminogen activator (rt-PA),[1] mostly in the treatment of acute myocardial infarction, provides a substantial amount of material on which to base an appraisal of 'risk' and 'benefit' with this powerful new thrombolytic agent. It is my purpose in this paper to assess the balance of clinical events associated with rt-PA, and to look at the fundamental question of whether a particular dosing scheme may minimize risk and yet maintain or even maximize benefit. I shall draw on published data for Genentech and Boehringer rt-PA as well as presenting some of the information gathered in Wellcome's international clinical trials programme with rt-PA. I shall deal specifically with the use of rt-PA in acute myocardial infarction.

The elements of risk and benefit with rt-PA treatment

The elements of risk and benefit for rt-PA are shown in Table 1. Risk with rt-PA seems to be concentrated in one area, that of unwanted haemorrhage.[1] Some risk of haemorrhage is common to all thrombolytic drugs.[1,2] rt-PA is a copy of a human protein and as such should not be antigenic in man; this has, thus far, proved to be the case. Concern has been stated that antigens derived from Chinese hamster ovary cells, the cells in which the gene for tissue plasminogen activator is expressed, may cause adverse reactions upon retreatment[2] but in the absence of any systematic study of retreatment with rt-PA such concern is conjectural. Benefit can be judged in a number of ways such as selective coronary arteriography to demonstrate lysis of intracoronary thrombi,[3–6] contrast or radionuclide left ventriculography to measure left ventricular size and/or function,[7–12] and tracking survival.[12,13] Lytic efficacy was the focus of attention in early studies

Table 1 *The elements of risk and benefit with use of rt-PA in the treatment of acute myocardial infarction.*

Risk	*Benefit*
Haemorrhage	Maximal lytic efficacy Minimal instability (reocclusion/reinfarction) Minimal extent of myocardial necrosis Preservation of left ventricular function Reduction in mortality

Table 2 *Data on efficacy and haemorrhagic complications from the European Cooperative Study Group's single-blind, randomized trial in acute myocardial infarction.*

Feature	rt-PA group			Streptokinase group		
	Patient numbers		*Percentage*	*Patient numbers*		*Percentage*
*Patency of infarct-related coronary artery at 75 to 90 minutes from start of treatment	43/62	=	69%	34/62	=	55%
Haematoma at catheter site	13/64	=	20%	22/65	=	34%
Prolonged bleeding at puncture site	4/64	=	6%	12/65	=	18%
Blood transfusion given	4/64	=	6%	5/65	=	8%

*Arteriographically demonstrated patency assessed by a grading scheme similar, but not identical, to the TIMI perfusion grading scheme.

Data taken from Tables III and IV of reference 3.

with rt-PA[1] and the single most often quoted measure has been patency of the infarct-related coronary artery, defined as a Thrombolysis In Myocardial Infarction (TIMI) perfusion grade[4] of 2 or 3, at 90 minutes after start of treatment. In similar manner arteriographic patency was used as the indicator of efficacy with the dose-finding work on Wellcome rt-PA in which, according to traditional drug development principles, the optimum balance between risk and benefit was sought.

General points on haemorrhagic risk, from published literature

Treatment of patients with intravenous rt-PA is associated with some risk of haemorrhage, as with all other thrombolytic drugs. Haemorrhagic complications are not unexpected when a powerful thrombolytic is administered to secure the swiftest possible lysis of an acutely occlusive coronary thrombus for it is inevitable that any concurrent protective haemostatic plugs will be subject to the circulating drug's destructive influence.[1] However some had hoped that the relative fibrin-selectivity of rt-PA, compared for example with streptokinase, and the fact that rt-PA engenders a relatively minor degree of systemic activation of the fibrinolytic system with consequent plasminaemia and hypofibrinogenaemia might mean less trouble from haemorrhage during and after treatment with rt-PA than with a non-fibrin-selective drug. Some measure of support for this view had been provided by the results of the European Cooperative Study Group's (ECSG) single-blind randomized trial of rt-PA versus streptokinase published in 1985.[3] The 43 patients randomized to rt-PA received an initial bolus of heparin 5000 IU followed by rt-PA 0.75 mg/kg over 90 minutes; the 34 patients randomized to streptokinase received the same initial bolus of heparin, plus methylprednisolone 250 mg and aspirin 500 mg, followed by streptokinase 1.5 MU over 60 minutes. Lytic efficacy was superior and bleeding complications less frequently encountered with rt-PA (Table 2), but numbers are small and the streptokinase group received aspirin whereas the rt-PA group did not. No such difference in haemorrhagic complications with rt-PA compared with streptokinase emerged in the detailed report[14] on that aspect of the TIMI Trial – Phase I, a double-blind randomized trial which showed marked superiority in lytic efficacy for rt-PA,[4] published in January 1988 (Table 3). The 143 patients randomized to rt-PA were given an initial bolus of heparin 5000 IU followed by rt-PA 80 mg over 3 hours (40 mg in first hour, 20 mg in second hour, 20 mg in third hour) and the 147 randomized to streptokinase were given the same initial bolus of heparin followed by streptokinase 1.5 MU over 1 hour; both groups also received intravenous heparin 1000 IU/hour beginning 3 hours after the initial bolus and subsequently adjusted to maintain the activated partial thromboplastin time at 1.5 to 2.0 times normal until pre-discharge cardiac catheterization 8 to 10 days later; aspirin was not used during this period.[4,14]

Thus in the larger TIMI-I trial, with some difference in the thrombolytic drug regimens and no concomitant aspirin for the rt-PA or streptokinase groups, haemorrhagic complications with rt-PA were similar to those with streptokinase. Moreover, the frequency of transfusions in the rt-PA and streptokinase groups was not significantly different (Table 3). In both the ECSG and TIMI-I trials all patients had acute coronary arteriography and, in keeping with the experience in other studies, most of the haemorrhages were at catheterization or other vascular puncture sites.

Minimizing haemorrhagic risk, particularly in terms of intracranial haemorrhage

With haemorrhage established as a risk, evidently the only significant risk, of treatment with rt-PA the obvious question is whether dosing adjustment can make any difference to that risk? Evidence suggesting that it can has come from the TIMI-II trial. In the open-label TIMI-II Pilot Study[15] there were five cases of intracranial haemorrhage among a total of 326 patients treated with 150 mg of the predominantly single-chain rt-PA (alteplase); 90 mg was given in the first hour with 10%

Table 3 *Data on efficacy and haemorrhagic complications from the Thrombolysis in Myocardial Infarction (TIMI) Trial – Phase I, a double-blind, randomized trial.*

	rt-PA group (n=143)			*Streptokinase group (n=147)*		
Feature	*Patient numbers*		*Percentage*	*Patient numbers*		*Percentage*
Reperfusion of infarct-related coronary artery at 75 to 90 minutes from start of treatment	70/113	=	62%	37/119	=	31%
Type of blood loss, at any site						
'Major'	22	=	15%	23	=	16%
'Minor' and 'loss at no site'	25	=	17%	23	=	16%
Blood loss at catheterization site						
'Major'	17	=	12%	16	=	11%
'Minor'	17	=	12%	17	=	12%
'Contributing'	5	=	3%	7	=	5%
Blood loss at other puncture sites						
'Major' and 'minor' and 'contributing'	7	=	5%	6	=	4%
Gastrointestinal blood loss						
'Major', 'minor' and 'contributing'	7	=	5%	10	=	4%
Frequency of blood transfusion associated with bleeding events	32	=	22%	29	=	20%

Data taken from reference 4 and Tables 2 and 3 of reference 14. See reference 14 for definitions of 'major', 'minor' and 'loss at no site'. 'Contributing' means that another site was the primary cause of blood loss, but this site with or without other sites probably contributed to the blood loss.

Table 4 *Intracranial haemorrhage in the TIMI-II Trial with two different doses of the same predominantly single-chain rt-PA.*

Part of trial from which data obtained	*Total dose of rt-PA over 6 hours*	*Patients treated*	*Intracranial haemorrhage*	
			Number	*Percentage*
Pilot open-label (E)	150 mg	326	5	1.5%
Main trial	150 mg	581	11	1.9%
Pooled open-label and main trial	150 mg	1014	16	1.6%
Main trial	100 mg	1311	7	0.5%
Pooled open-label and main trial	100 mg	1452	8	0.6%

Data taken from Table 1 of reference 17.

as an initial bolus, 20 mg in the second hour, and 10 mg/hour in the remaining 4 hours. Heparin was started with a bolus at the same time as rt-PA infusion was commenced and aspirin was begun on day 2. Three of the five episodes of intracranial haemorrhage occurred during the first 24 hours and three were fatal. On the basis of this frequency of intracranial haemorrhage of 1.5% the TIMI Operations Committee instructed that the rt-PA dose for the remainder of the TIMI-II trial should be reduced to 100 mg over 6 hours (60 mg in the first hour with 10% as an initial bolus, 20 mg in the second hour, and 5 mg/hour in the remaining 4 hours).[16]

When the preliminary results of the experience with the 100 mg dose of rt-PA in TIMI-II, as of June 1987, were published in October 1987[17] it could be seen that 1311 patients had received the 100 mg dose and there had been seven cases of intracranial haemorrhage (7/1311 = 0.5%) whereas among 581 patients in the first part of the main TIMI-II trial who had received the 150 mg dose there had been 11 cases of intracranial haemorrhage (11/581 = 1.9%). Pooling the results for all TIMI open-label and main trial patients treated with 150 mg of rt-PA showed 16 cases of intracranial haemorrhage among 1014 patients (16/1014 = 1.6%); in comparison, similarly pooled data on 1452 patients treated with 100mg of the same predominantly single-chain rt-PA over 6 hours showed eight cases of intracranial haemorrhage (8/1452 = 0.6%). These data are shown in Table 4. The Genentech data sheet for rt-PA now specifically states that 'a dose of 150 mg of ACTIVASE® should not be used because it has been associated with an increase in intracranial bleeding'. Thus, for the infrequent but clinically very serious complication of intracranial haemorrhage after treatment with rt-PA it was concluded on the basis of relatively small numbers of events that the higher dose (150 mg) was more hazardous than a lower dose (100 mg). But doubts remain. Are these results two points on a dose–response line or curve, is there a threshold for more intracranial bleeding somewhere between the 100 mg and 150 mg dose of rt-PA, or are results a quirk of small numbers and therefore spurious?

Stroke in acute myocardial infarction

Stroke is a recognized complication of acute myocardial infarction,[18–20] in most cases probably of embolic or thrombotic aetiology. Therefore strokes that occur in patients treated with

Table 5 *Data on stroke in two large double-blind, randomized trials of thrombolytic treatment in acute myocardial infarction.*

	Treatment Subgroup		
Study and clinical event	*rt-PA*	*Placebo*	*Streptokinase*
ASSET, stroke, up to 1 month			
'Haemorrhagic'	7	2	
'Embolic'	11	17	
'Unclassified'	10	6	
Total (percentage)	28 (1.1%)	25 (1.0%)	
ISIS-2, stroke, in hospital			
'Confirmed haemorrhagic'		0	7
'Other, day 0–1'		13	20
'Other, after day 1'		54	34
Total (percentage)		67 (0.8%)	61 (0.7%)

Data taken for ASSET taken from reference 13 and for ISIS-2 from reference 21.

thrombolytic therapy are not necessarily *caused by* thrombolytic therapy. The reported incidence of stroke varies, depending on the criteria for diagnosis and other methodological details. In three studies of stroke during the hospital course after admission with acute myocardial infarction the incidence was 13/783 (= 1.7%),[18] 18/740 (= 2.4%)[19] and 14/1277 (= 1.1%).[20] Thrombolytic therapy might possibly reduce the number of strokes caused by emboli of cardiac origin. In the Anglo-Scandinavian Study of Early Thrombolysis (ASSET)[13] embolic strokes were separately identified, and occurred in 11 patients treated with rt-PA (11/2512=0.4%) and 17 treated with placebo (17/2493 = 0.7%). There is, however, concern about the risk of haemorrhagic stroke being enhanced by thrombolytic therapy. Heparin could also augment that risk. Some data for rt-PA from ASSET[13] and for streptokinase from the Second International Study of Infarct Survival (ISIS-2)[21] are of interest in this context and are shown in Table 5. Heparin was used routinely in the first 24 hours in ASSET but not in ISIS-2. Haemorrhagic stroke was indeed more common in the patients treated with active thrombolytic therapy than in those treated with placebo in both trials. However an excess of embolic stroke in those receiving placebo in ASSET and of strokes not confirmed as haemorrhagic after day 1 in ISIS-2 resulted in total numbers of strokes in active and placebo treatment groups in both studies which were not significantly different. Thus with specific reference to rt-PA, as used with concomitant heparin in a fairly large trial,[13] it seems that the overall risk of stroke is not significantly increased compared with the risk with heparin alone. Moreover the percentage stroke rates in the two treatment subgroups are very close indeed to the stroke rate in one of the recently published studies of stroke associated with acute myocardial infarction where thrombolytic therapy was not used and heparin anticoagulation was administered only to patients thought to be at high risk of thrombosis.[20]

In a review focusing on intracranial haemorrhage with thrombolytic therapy Tiefenbrunn and Ludbrook commented that 'The results available suggest that any increment in intracranial bleeding that might be ascribed to treatment with a lytic agent in myocardial infarction is small and offset by a decrease in the incidence of thromboembolic stroke'.[22]

To return to the TIMI-II Pilot Study data. Are there any clues as to why the 5 patients with intracranial haemorrhage should have suffered this complication? Brief case histories are given in one paper.[15] The patients' ages were 69, 62, 52, 67, and 66 years – mostly somewhat above the mean age of 57 years for the whole subgroup of patients who received the 150 mg dose of rt-PA. Most thrombolytic studies, with the notable exception of ISIS-2, have an upper age-limit of 70 or 75 years. In two papers reporting stroke after myocardial infarction the mean ages of the patients who suffered strokes were 64.6 years[18] and 65.6 years.[19] There are no data on the patients' weights so the dose of rt-PA per unit body weight cannot be ascertained. One patient was later discovered to have a history of one episode of transient neurological symptoms, one had suffered a stroke 15 years earlier and had been treated for hypertension, and two others were also on treatment for hypertension. This raises the whole question of exclusion criteria for rt-PA treatment. Many investigators have excluded patients with a history of stroke, as we have done and continue to do in Wellcome trials. And what of transient cerebral ischaemic attacks? Our inclination at the moment is to exclude patients with such a history. There is fairly general agreement that patients with high blood pressure, say $\geqslant$ 180 or 200 mmHg systolic or $\geqslant$ 110 or 120 mmHg diastolic, at the time of consideration for rt-PA treatment should be excluded. But the question that still needs clarification concerns the risk associated with treated hypertension and a fairly normal blood pressure at the time of presentation with acute myocardial infarction. The more stringent and extensive the exclusion criteria, the fewer are the benefits from rt-PA but presumably the more favourable will the adverse events profile appear.

Dosing rt-PA with reference to body weight

I turn now to the question of weight-adjusted dosing of rt-PA. Unlike the pattern in TIMI-I[4] and TIMI-II,[15,23,24] in which a fixed dose of rt-PA was used, some investigators (for example, the ECSG[3] and the Thrombolysis and Angioplasty in Myocardial Infarction (TAMI) Study Group[25]) have used a dose-by-weight approach. The TAMI Group were able to compare their experience in 178 patients given 150 mg of rt-PA of predominantly single-chain form over 8 hours (60 mg in first hour with 10% as an initial bolus, then 20 mg/hour for 2 hours, then 10 mg/hour for 5 hours – Group A regimen) and a subsequent group of 208 patients given the same total dose of 150 mg of rt-PA but administered using a weight-adjusted scheme and a shorter maintenance infusion (1 mg/kg in the first hour with 10% as an initial bolus and a maximum dose of 90 mg, and the remainder of the 150 mg over the next 5 hours – Group B regimen).[25] Heparin was started during the first hour and continued for at least 3 days, and aspirin and dipyridamole were also given. The infarct-artery patency at coronary arteriography 94 ± 30 minutes into treatment was 64% in Group A versus 75% in Group B ($p = 0.02$) and reocclusion was demonstrated at 7 to 10 days in 17% of Group A versus 13% of Group B patients ($p = 0.35$). Bleeding was reduced in Group B patients, as evidenced by a decrease in requirement for ⩾ 2 units of packed red blood cells (36% in Group A versus 27% in Group B, $p = 0.05$) and lower incidence of gastrointestinal bleeding (12% in Group A versus 4% in Group B, $p = 0.002$). Perhaps surprisingly the only two intracranial haemorrhages in the whole study were in Group B patients; this highlights the need for relatively large studies (probably at least 1000 per treatment group) before conclusions can be drawn concerning the relative incidence of rather infrequent events. The results of this sequential open comparison by the TAMI Group hinted at less haemorrhagic risk with superior lytic efficacy when a dose-by-weight approach for rt-PA treatment was used. The ECSG, however, have moved away from the dose-by-weight approach of their trial published in 1985:[3] in their latest double-blind, randomized, placebo-controlled trial with 355 patients allocated to receive rt-PA, a fixed dose (60 mg in first hour with 10 mg as initial bolus, and 20 mg/hour for 2 hours) was used.[12]

In the recently presented overview[26] of haemorrhagic risk in 810 consecutive patients with acute myocardial infarction entered into TAMI Studies, 561 of whom had been treated with rt-PA, 102 with urokinase, and 147 with a combination of the two thrombolytic agents, lighter weight ($p < 0.01$) was found to be among the most important risk factors. Body weight deserves close attention in the light of accumulating trial evidence. It can readily be taken into consideration by the physician and nursing staff involved in the management of patients with acute myocardial infarction.

Wellcome's experience in trials with its double-chain rt-PA

Some interesting points have emerged in Wellcome's clinical trials work with a double-chain rt-PA (duteplase). Doses are expressed in megaunits (1 MU = 1×10^6 IU) of activity, referenced to the international t-PA standard which is a melanoma-derived t-PA; at the time of our earlier trials we used a kinetic chromogenic assay and more recently a clot lysis assay.

Dose-ranging and duration-of-dose studies

The main elements of our dose-ranging work with rt-PA were two studies, designated P52-10[27] and P52-03,[28] carried out in the USA. Their key features are shown in Tables 6 and 7. Patients were eligible for inclusion in these studies if they were of age ⩽ 75 years, had experienced cardiac ischaemic-type chest pain of duration at least 30 min but less than 6 hours, and had

Table 6 *Main elements of the P52-01 open study of Wellcome rt-PA in acute myocardial infarction.*

Age $\leqslant$ 75 years
Chest pain of duration $\geqslant$ 30 minutes but < 6 hours
Electrocardiogram showing ST segment elevation $\geqslant$ 0.2 mV into two standard leads or $\geqslant$ 0.3 mV in at least two precordial leads
No contraindications (standard set for thrombolytic therapy)
Immediate treatment with a range of rt-PA 'lytic' doses over 90 minutes, with heparin 5000 IU given after arterial sheath placed
Coronary arteriography at 90 minutes from start of rt-PA
'Responders' continue with 'maintenance' rt-PA at one third of initial rate for 90 minutes
Heparin infusion continued to end of study period at 72 hours, with infusion rate adjusted to keep activated partial thromboplastin time at 2.0 to 2.5 times control

Table 7 *Additional details of the P52-03 open study of Wellcome rt-PA in acute myocardial infarction.*

As for P52-01, but:
Specified 'lytic' dose of rt-PA over 90 minutes
Several maintenance infusions tested, with durations 4.5 to 24 hours
Repeat coronary arteriography at 12 to 24 hours
Heparin stopped at 72 hours
End of study period at 96 hours

electrocardiographic ST segment elevation of $\geqslant$ 0.2 mV in two standard leads or $\geqslant$ 0.3 mV in at least two precordial leads. Exclusion criteria were very similar to those in most published trials of rt-PA. Treatment with rt-PA was commenced as quickly as possible, usually in the Emergency Room, and the patient was taken to the cardiac catheterization laboratory so that coronary arteriograms could be filmed at 90 minutes after start of rt-PA treatment. Heparin, 5000 IU as a bolus, was given after the arterial sheath had been inserted and continued for 72 hours in all patients with documented perfusion (TIMI grades 2 or 3) of the infarct artery to maintain the activated partial thromboplastin time at 2.0 to 2.5 times normal.

In our P52-01 lytic efficacy study a range of doses of rt-PA was administered over 90 minutes. As described by Goldberg when he presented preliminary data at the 60th Scientific Sessions of the American Heart Association in November 1987, the response rate ('Responders' are those with TIMI perfusion grades 2 or 3 for the infarct-related coronary artery – see Table 8) varied with dose of rt-PA administered.[27] The pattern was that of a dose-response relationship with increasing doses per unit body weight. Haemorrhagic complications were analysed according to dosing intervals for dose of rt-PA administered per unit body weight, with meticulous attention having been paid to recording all haemorrhagic events – even minor oozing at a vascular puncture site. The level of seriousness assigned to a particular haemorrhagic event is indicated in Table 9. There appeared to be a dose-dependent relationship between the total dose of rt-PA and

Table 8 *The evaluation of lytic efficacy in early clinical trials with Wellcome rt-PA in acute myocardial infarction.*

Lytic efficacy	Judged by selective coronary arteriography 'Responders' are those with TIMI perfusion grade of 2 or 3 for infarct-related artery 'Non-responders' are those with TIMI perfusion grade of 0 or 1 for infarct-related artery

Table 9 *Points considered in assigning a level of seriousness to a haemorrhagic complication in clinical trials with Wellcome rt-PA in acute myocardial infarction.*

Seriousness	Not serious Inconsequential, not affecting clinical status Serious Severe enough to need transfusion and/or affect clinical status Life-threatening Intracranial haemorrhage Haemopericardium with tamponade Haemorrhage with haemodynamic compromise Fatal haemorrhagic complication

haemorrhage.[27] Further interim analysis of the accumulating data in this study since Goldberg's presentation has confirmed the initial impression that this relationship is stronger for 'Serious and Life-threatening bleeding' ($p = 0.005$) than for 'Any bleeding' ($p = 0.190$). The contribution of weight to haemorrhagic complications was also analysed in a stepwise logistic regression model, asking the specific question 'Controlling for total dose in MU, does weight contribute significantly to bleeding?' The result is that for a given total dose of rt-PA a lighter patient has a significantly higher chance of developing 'Serious or Life-threatening bleeding' than does a heavier patient.

The data from our P52-01 study confirmed the ability of Wellcome rt-PA to achieve patency rates for the infarct-related coronary artery of the same order as reported by other investigators with other forms of rt-PA. Since both efficacy and haemorrhagic complications appeared to be dose-related, it was felt that administration of rt-PA on a dose-by-weight basis might optimize the risk : benefit ratio.[27]

The objectives of our P52-03 study were to acquire further data on efficacy of Wellcome rt-PA by coronary arteriographic assessment at the end of a 90-minute lytic dose; to explore the possible benefit of a prolonged maintenance infusion in preventing early reocclusion; and to assess whether there is increased risk associated with a prolonged maintenance infusion. Some of the results were presented by Thadani at the 61st Scientific Session of the American Heart Association in November 1988.[28] The lytic infusion of rt-PA was given at one of two dose levels (0.20 or 0.28 MU/kg/hour, clot lysis units of t-PA activity) for 90 minutes and among 207 assessable patients the Responders numbered 134 (134/207 = 65%). The assigned maintenance dosing scheme and technically satisfactory second coronary arteriogram, according to protocol, were completed in 117 of the 134 Responders; data

Table 10 *Clinical events in the first 882 patients with acute myocardial infarction treated with the International Dose (weight-adjusted) of Wellcome rt-PA.*

Events	*Patient numbers (out of total of 882 patients)*	*Percentage*
In-hospital mortality	43	4.9%
Transfusion (exclusive of surgery)	34	3.9%
Intracranial haemorrhage		
Fatal	1	0.1%
Non-fatal	3	0.3%
Retroperitoneal haemorrhage	2	0.2%
*Allergic reaction	2	0.2%
Left ventricular rupture	4	0.5%
Ventricular septal defect	3	0.3%
Electromechanical dissociation (pathology not known)	7	0.8%

*Not necessarily to rt-PA; patients received radiographic contrast for coronary arteriography.

were therefore available on 117 patients who had been randomized to one of four maintenance dosing groups (0.012, 0.024, 0.036 and 0.048 MU/kg/hour, clot lysis units of t-PA activity). Reocclusion rates at 12 to 24 hours were similar for the four dosing groups, overall being 13.7%. This study demonstrated that infarct-related coronary arteries were sometimes reoccluding even when there was no rt-PA-free interval before the second coronary arteriogram.

Work by Gold and colleagues in Boston indicated apparent benefit in terms of reducing the reocclusion rate with 4-hour maintenance infusions of rt-PA following initial 90-minute lytic infusions,[29,30] but investigators in Europe had found no differences in arteriographically demonstrated coronary reocclusion between a 6-hour maintenance infusion of rt-PA or placebo.[31] Although data are conflicting on the efficacy of maintenance infusions of rt-PA relative to the issue of reocclusion, it was the case that haemorrhagic complications categorized as 'Serious or Life-threatening' increased with increasing dose of rt-PA in our P52-03 study. This issue was explored further in a presentation made at the 38th Annual Scientific Session of the American College of Cardiology in March 1989.[32] Our results prompt consideration of at least two possibilities concerning the role of maintenance infusions of rt-PA. First, should we have used higher doses in the hope of reducing further our reocclusion rates? This would seem unwise on the basis of our safety data, for higher doses will exact a penalty in terms of increased 'Serious and Life-threatening bleeding'. Second, are shorter maintenance infusions worth pursuing? On the safety level this approach seems promising, but how short should the maintenance phase be? The Genentech and Boehringer recommended dosing scheme for rt-PA is a lytic dose of 60 mg in the first hour, of which 6 to 10 mg is administered as an initial bolus, and then 20 mg/hour for 2 hours as a maintenance dose. Wellcome's choice for the new efficacy and safety trials for rt-PA which were conducted after the P52-01 and P52-03 studies was to test the dose-by-weight approach with a lytic dose chosen to give standard efficacy (that is, coronary patency of around 70% at 90 minutes) and a total dose likely to result in a fairly low (< 10%) incidence of 'Serious or Life-threatening' haemorrhagic complications in the context of acute cardiac catheterization procedures. We opted for a 1-hour lytic plus 3-hour maintenance regimen. The precise dosing instructions were to administer the rt-PA at a dose of 0.40 MU/kg in the first hour, with 10% of that dose as an initial bolus, and to follow with 0.20 MU/kg over 3 hours. We continued to use concomitant heparin, but realized that there is no clear and convincing evidence of its value in enhancing the efficacy of rt-PA without compromising safety. A small study has since been reported by the TAMI Study Group[33] indicating that heparin does not appear to have an important facilitative effect on rt-PA-mediated coronary clot lysis, nor does it seem to increase haemorrhagic complications. The data on rt-PA with or without heparin from the ISIS-3 trial will be of great interest.

Lytic efficacy and safety with a weight-adjusted dosing scheme

Our results in more than six hundred patients now treated with Wellcome rt-PA on the weight-adjusted regimen have fulfilled our expectations in the sense that we are achieving efficacy, as judged by 90-minute patency of the infarct-related coronary artery, close to the 70% mark. The first presentation of efficacy and safety data on some of these patients was made recently.[34] In a study currently evaluating reocclusion at 24 to 48 hours from start of rt-PA treatment the preliminary results support a reocclusion rate less than half of that found in the prolonged infusion P52-03 study. The safety profile is outlined in Table 10, which lists selected clinical events in the first 882 patients with acute myocardial infarction treated with this regimen. The in-hospital mortality of 4.9%, non-surgical transfusion rate of 3.9% and incidence of intracranial haemorrhage of 0.4% are all encouraging figures in comparison with other published studies.

Concluding comments

It seems inevitable that some risk of haemorrhage will attend the use of thrombolytic therapy to achieve lysis of obstructive intra-coronary thrombi, for extracardiac haemostatic plugs will also be subject to lysis.[1,22,35] It is therefore of paramount importance to evaluate each thrombolytic drug developed for clinical use in terms of both safety and efficacy. Special attention must be given to clinically significant haemorrhagic complications such as those within the compass of 'Serious or Life-threatening bleeding'. The clinician should expect clear characterization of risk and benefit features for all thrombolytic drugs that are licensed. Any factor that optimizes the risk: benefit ratio should be identified.[35] At present a dose-by-weight approach for rt-PA is the only measure that holds promise of optimizing the ratio. Wellcome's experience suggests it is an approach that can yield satisfactory results. As new dosing schemes for rt-PA are explored[36,37] the debate over whether or not to test weight-adjusted regimens will presumably continue. The apparently widespread inclination among clinicians, on both sides of the Atlantic, to extrapolate from the favourable results for aspirin in ISIS-2, and therefore to use aspirin as adjunctive therapy with rt-PA, has made it more or less essential to incorporate aspirin into the design of most new trials of rt-PA. The safety of rt-PA with heparin and aspirin has not been fully established. It is appropriate, however, to proceed with caution for in one study[12] there were five cases of intracranial haemorrhage within the first 3 days of treatment with rt-PA among 355 patients (1.4%). Patency and especially reocclusion may be influenced by this adjunctive use of aspirin with rt-PA. The optimum rt-PA regimen may also depend on the presence of aspirin. Aspirin may have a better effect as an adjunct to thrombolytic therapy in patients who present early after onset of symptoms.[38] There is still scope for a great deal of clinical research to ascertain the best management schemes for patients who present with acute myocardial infarction requiring thrombolytic therapy, so that risk and benefit can be balanced to advantage.

Acknowledgements

I thank Dr Judy LittleJohn and other members of the tPA Project Group, Division of Clinical Research, Burroughs Wellcome Co, Research Triangle Park, North Carolina, USA for help in the preparation of this manuscript and acknowledge the contribution of the clinical investigators and research co-ordinators of the Burroughs Wellcome t-PA Study Group in carrying out the P52-01 and P52-03 studies to which I have referred.

References

1. Loscalzo J, Braunwald E, Tissue plasminogen activator. *N. Engl. J. Med. 319*, 1988, 925–931.
2. Sherry S, Recombinant tissue plasminogen activator (rt-PA): is it the thrombolytic agent of choice for an evolving acute myocardial infarction? *Am. J. Cardiol. 59*, 1987, 984–989.
3. Verstraete M, Bory M, Collen D, *et al.*, Randomised trial of intravenous recombinant tissue-type plasminogen activator versus intravenous streptokinase in acute myocardial infarction: report from the European Cooperative Study Group for Recombinant Tissue-type Plasminogen Activator. *Lancet 1*, 1985, 842–847.
4. Chesebro J H, Knatterud G, Roberts R, *et al.*, Thrombolysis in Myocardial Infarction (TIMI) Trial, Phase I: a comparison between intravenous tissue plasminogen activator and intravenous streptokinase: clinical findings through hospital discharge. *Circulation 76*, 1987, 142–154.
5. Topol E J, Morris D C, Smalling R W, *et al.*, A multicenter, randomized, placebo-controlled trial of a new form of intravenous recombinant tissue-type plasminogen activator (Activase) in acute myocardial infarction. *J. Am. Coll. Cardiol. 9*, 1987, 1205–1213.
6. National Heart Foundation of Australia Coronary Thrombolysis Group. Coronary thrombolysis and myocardial salvage by tissue plasminogen activator given up to 4 hours after onset of myocardial infarction. *Lancet 1*, 1988, 203–208.
7. Guerci A D, Gerstenblith G, Brinker J A, *et al.*, A randomized trial of intravenous tissue plasminogen activator for acute myocardial infarction with subsequent randomization to elective coronary angioplasty. *N. Engl. J. Med. 317*, 1987, 1613–1618.
8. Sheehan F H, Determinants of improved left ventricular function after thrombolytic therapy in acute myocardial infarction. *J. Am. Coll. Cardiol. 9* 1987, 937–944.
9. O'Rourke M, Baron D, Keogh R, *et al.*, Limitation of myocardial infarction by early infusion of recombinant tissue-type plasminogen activator. *Circulation 77*, 1988, 1311–1315.
10. Norris R M, White H D, Therapeutic trials in coronary thrombosis should measure left ventricular function as primary end-point of treatment. *Lancet 1*, 1988, 104–106.
11. Armstrong P W, Baigrie R S, Daly P A, *et al.*, Tissue Plasminogen Activator: Toronto (TPAT) placebo-controlled randomized trial in acute myocardial infarction. *J. Am. Coll. Cardiol. 13*, 1989, 1469–1476.
12. Van de Werf F, Arnold A E R, Intravenous tissue plasminogen activator and size of infarct, left ventricular function, and survival in acute myocardial infarction. *Br. Med. J.* 297, 1988, 1374–1379.
13. Wilcox R G, von der Lippe G, Olsson C G, Jensen G, Skene A M, Hampton J R, Trial of tissue plasminogen activator for mortality reduction in acute myocardial infarction: Anglo-Scandinavian Study of Early Thrombolysis (ASSET). *Lancet 2*, 1988, 525–530.

14. Rao A K, Pratt C, Berke A, *et al.*, Thrombolysis in myocardial infarction (TIMI) Trial – Phase I: hemorrhagic manifestations and changes in plasma fibrinogen and the fibrinolytic system in patients treated with recombinant tissue plasminogen activator and streptokinase. *J.Am.Coll.Cardiol. 11*, 1988, 1–11.
15. Passamani E, Hodges M, Herman M, *et al.*, The Thrombolysis in Myocardial Infarction (TIMI) Phase II Pilot Study: tissue plasminogen activator followed by percutaneous transluminal coronary angioplasty. *J.Am.Coll.Cardiol. 10*, 1987, 51B 64B.
16. TIMI Operations Committee: Braunwald E, Knatterud G L, Passamani E, Announcement of protocol change in Thrombolysis in Myocardial Infarction trial (Letter to the Editor). *J.Am.Coll.Cardiol. 9*, 1987, 467.
17. TIMI Operations Committee: Braunwald E, Knatterud G L, Passamani E, Robertson T L, Solomon R, Update from the Thrombolysis in Myocardial Infarction trial (Letter to the Editor). *J.Am.Coll.Cardiol. 10*, 1987, 970.
18. Thompson P L, Robinson J S, Stroke after acute myocardial infarction: relation to infarct size. *Br.Med.J. 2*, 1978, 457–459.
19. Komrad M S, Coffey E, Coffey K S, McKinnis R, Massey E W, Califf R M, Myocardial infarction and stroke. *Neurology 34*, 1984, 1403–1409.
20. Puletti M, Morocutti C, Tronca M, *et al.*, Cerebrovascular accidents in acute myocardial infarction. *Ital.J.Neurol.Sci. 8*, 1987, 245–248.
21. ISIS-2 (Second International Study of Infarct Survival) Collaborative Group. Randomised trial of intravenous streptokinase, oral aspirin, both or neither among 17,187 cases of suspected acute myocardial infarction: ISIS-2. *Lancet 2*, 1988, 349–360.
22. Tiefenbrunn A J, Ludbrook P A, Coronary thrombolysis – it's worth the risk. *JAMA 261*, 1989, 2107–2108.
23. TIMI Research Group, Immediate vs delayed catheterization and angioplasty following thrombolytic therapy for acute myocardial infarction: TIMI II A results. *JAMA 260*, 1988, 2849–2858.
24. TIMI Study Group, Comparison of invasive and conservative strategies after treatment with intravenous tissue plasminogen activator in acute myocardial infarction: results of Thrombolysis in Myocardial Infarction (TIMI) Phase II Trial. *N.Engl.J.Med. 320*, 1989, 618–627.
25. Topol E J, George B S, Kereiakes D J, *et al.*, Comparison of two dose regimens of intravenous tissue plasminogen activator for acute myocardial infarction. *Am.J.Cardiol. 61*, 1988, 723–728.
26. Califf R M, Stump D, Topol E J, *et al.*, Overview of bleeding risk from the TAMI trials: two agents are better than one (Abstract). *J.Am.Coll.Cardiol. 13*, 1989, 198A.
27. Goldberg S, Turi Z, Efficacy and complications of recombinant double chain tissue plasminogen activator for acute myocardial infarction; results of a multicenter trial (Abstract). *Circulation 76* (Supplement IV), 1987, IV–305.
28. Thadani U, Reocclusion rate after prolonged infusion of double-chain tissue plasminogen activator in acute myocardial infarction (Abstract). *Circulation 78* (Supplement II), 1988, II–276.
29. Gold H K, Leinbach R C, Garabedian H D, *et al.*, Acute coronary reocclusion after thrombolysis with recombinant human tissue-type plasminogen activator: prevention by a maintenance infusion. *Circulation 73*, 1986, 347–352.
30. Johns J A, Gold H K, Leinbach R C, *et al.*, Prevention of coronary artery reocclusion and reduction in late coronary artery stenosis after thrombolytic therapy in patients with acute myocardial infarction: a randomized study of maintenance infusion of recombinant human tissue-type plasminogen activator. *Circulation 78*, 1988, 546–556.

31. Verstraete M, Arnold A E R, Brower R W, *et al.*, Acute coronary thrombolysis with recombinant human tissue-type plasminogen activator: initial patency and influence of maintained infusion on reocclusion rate. *Am.J.Cardiol. 60*, 1987, 231–237.
32. Thadani U, Bleeding complications after double-chain tPA: influence of dose and duration of infusion (Abstract). *J.Am.Coll.Cardiol. 13*, 1989, 77A.
33. Topol E J, George B S, Kereiakes D J, *et al.*, A randomized controlled trial of intravenous tissue plasminogen activator and early intravenous heparin in acute myocardial infarction. *Circulation 79*, 1989, 281–286.
34. Grines C L, Efficacy and safety of weight adjusted dosing of a new tissue plasminogen activator preparation in acute myocardial infarction (Abstract). *Circulation 78* (Supplement II), 1988, II–127.
35. Califf R M, Topol E J, George B S, *et al.*, Hemorrhagic complications associated with the use of intravenous tissue plasminogen activator in treatment of acute myocardial infarction. *Am.J.Med. 85*, 1988, 353–359.
36. Neuhaus K L, Feuerer W, Tebbe U, Jeep-Tebbe S, Vogt A, Efficacy of a 90-minute infusion of 100 mg tissue plasminogen activator (rt-PA) in acute myocardial infarction (Abstract). *Eur. Heart. J. 9* (Abstr. Supplement I), 1988, 9.
37. Schumacher R R, Smalling R W, Morris D C, Grossbard E B, A multicenter, randomized comparison of two doses of recombinant tissue plasminogen activator in treatment of myocardial infarction. *Circulation 78* (Supplement II), 1988, II–275.
38. Basinski A, Naylor C D, Aspirin and fibrinolysis (Letter to the Editor). *Lancet 2*, 1988, 1188–1189.

Chapter 7

MONOTHERAPY AND COMBINATION THERAPIES WITH PRO-UROKINASE, UROKINASE AND TISSUE PLASMINOGEN ACTIVATOR

Victor Gurewich

Tufts University School of Medicine, Boston, MA, USA

Introduction – Fibrin specific and non-specific fibrinolysis

When the endogenous fibrinolytic system is stimulated by non-pharmacological means such as exercise,[1] tourniquet occlusion,[2] or death,[3] accelerated fibrinolysis without accompanying fibrinogenolysis takes place. Thus, the hallmark of physiological fibrinolysis, mediated by endogenous activators, is fibrin specificity. By contrast, pharmacological fibrinolysis by streptokinase (SK) or urokinase (UK) is non-specific being accompanied by systemic plasminogen activation. Since plasmin is an enzyme with broad specificity, systemic plasminogen activation results in widespread proteolytic effects which include degradation of certain clotting factors (I, V, VII, XII), proteolysis of certain constituents of platelet and basement membrane, and activation of the complement pathway through activation of C1, C3 and C5.

The most obvious consequence of plasminemia is that hemostasis is compromised, not only as a result of degradation of important clotting factors, but also because of the generation of fibrinogen degradation products which interfere with platelet aggregation and fibrin polymerization[4] and which may enhance vascular permeability.[5] These effects of plasmin may be responsible for the high incidence of hemorrhagic myocardial infarction which Waller *et al.*[6] showed were associated with thrombolytic therapy with either SK or t-PA, but not with reperfusion induced by angioplasty. Paradoxically, plasmin has also been shown by Niewiarowski *et al.*[7] to induce platelet aggregation and the platelet release reaction, a phenomenon which may help explain certain clot promoting effects of SK and UK observed in experimental studies by Godal *et al.*[8] and Hirsh *et al.*[9] This pro-thrombotic plasmin effect may contribute to rethrombosis, an event which seriously compromises coronary thrombolytic therapy. One more effect of plasmin should be noted. The activation of certain complement zymogens results in the release of anaphylotoxins which were shown by Bennett *et al.* to be present in high concentrations in the blood of patients undergoing thrombolytic therapy.[10] Since anaphylotoxins induce tissue necrosis, their release during therapeutic thrombolysis may compromise myocardial salvage.

These deleterious effects of non-specific plasminogen activation have made the fibrin specific properties of the natural plasminogen activators attractive. The endogenous plasminogen activators, t-PA and pro-UK, achieve their fibrin specificity by activating only fibrin-bound plasminogen (for review see reference 11). However, at the high doses required for effective coronary thrombolysis by monotherapy with either t-PA or pro-UK, non-specific activation of plasma plasminogen takes place. At lower fibrin-specific doses, each activator is relatively ineffective. By contrast, when t-PA and pro-UK are combined, effective and fibrin specific clot lysis occurs.[12,13]

The clinical importance of fibrin specificity in therapeutic thrombolysis, though theoretically compelling, has not been established since no clinical trials comparing a fibrin specific regimen with non-specific thrombolysis have been conducted. It may be postulated, however, that fibrin specific thrombolysis will limit bleeding complications by preserving the hemostatic function, though this has been challenged.[14] In addition, fibrin specificity may enhance thrombolytic efficacy by conserving the normal reservoir of plasminogen and improve myocardial salvage by curtailing the compromising effects of interstitial hemorrhage and release of tissue necrosing substances.

Finally, all of the plasminogen activators have different mechanisms of action. As a result, different clinical indications may exist for certain activators or combination of activators. In this review, the properties and mechanism of action of pro-UK will be compared with those of UK and of t-PA.

A comparison of the thrombolytic properties of pro-UK and t-PA

Pro-urokinase was first isolated because of its selective binding to fibrin/Celite in urine.[15, 16] Since it was this property alone which led to the discovery of this novel form of UK, it was assumed that pro-UK had a similar fibrin clot affinity to that of t-PA. Surprisingly, this assumption turned out to be incorrect.[17] It became apparent that certain properties of fibrin/Celite and of urine were essential for binding. As a result, in a plasma milieu little or no binding of pro-UK to a fibrin clot was found. Nevertheless, despite its low affinity for a fibrin clot, pro-UK was shown to induce fibrin specific clot lysis in plasma *in vitro* and *in vivo*.[18, 19] The explanation for this phenomenon has been ascribed to a conformational change in plasminogen which takes place when it binds to fibrin.[17] Alternatively, it has been proposed by Lijnen *et al.*[20] that dissociation of a pro-UK: inhibitor complex in plasma is triggered by fibrin. However, no such inhibitor has yet been identified. Regardless of the mechanism, all investigators agree that pro-UK is stable in plasma for extended periods, and in contrast to UK, does not form SDS-stable complexes.[17] As a result, the fibrinolytic properties of pro-UK when incubated for several days in plasma remain uncompromised[18] and plasma plasminogen remains intact.[21]

This zymogenic property distinguishes pro-UK from t-PA. The latter is active, both in its single and its two-chain forms and consequently has a relatively short t1/2 to inhibition in plasma. Tissue plasminogen activator is inactivated by several plasma inhibitors which include PAI-1, C1-esterase inhibitor, α2-antiplasmin and α2-macroglobulin. Most of the circulating t-PA intrinsic to plasma is in the form of a complex with PAI-1.[22] In natural fibrinolysis, t-PA evades inhibition

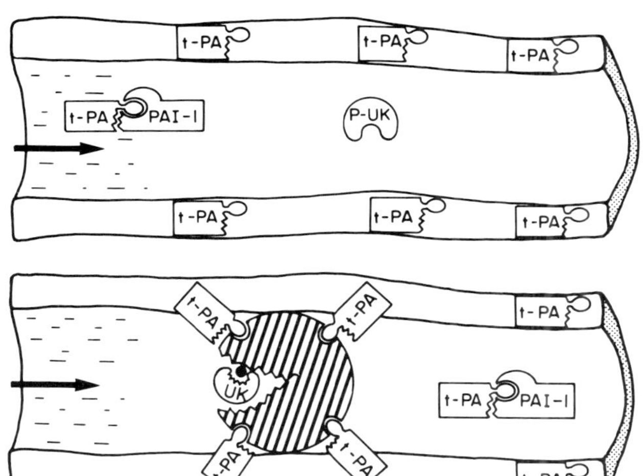

Figure 1A *Some elements of physiological fibrinolysis by t-PA and pro-UK. As illustrated above, t-PA is stored in the vessel and circulates in blood largely as a complex with the inhibitor, PAI-I. By contrast, pro-UK is found intact in blood. As illustrated below, when a thrombus forms, t-PA is released locally, binds to fibrin and initiates fibrinolysis. The partially degraded clot is then further lysed by pro-UK which is activated to UK on the clot surface as shown.*

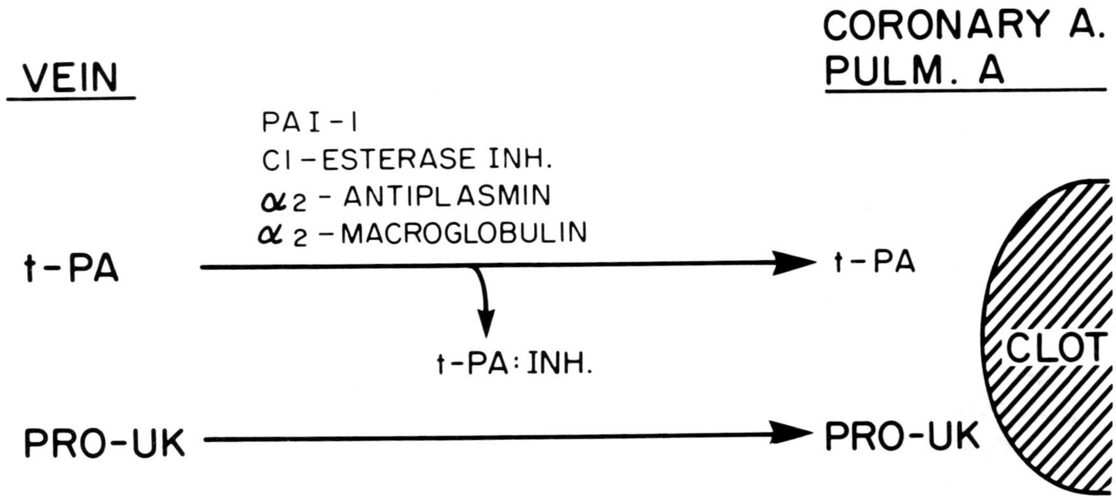

Figure 1B *Pharmacological fibrinolysis by t-PA and pro-UK. When t-PA is given intravenously, its access to a remote thrombus is attenuated by inhibitors which are consumed in the process. Only the uncomplexed t-PA binds to the fibrin thrombus where it resists inhibition. By contrast, since pro-UK is zygomenic in plasma, its passage to the clot is not attenuated by inhibitors and inhibitors are not consumed*

because it is released from the vessel wall at the site of a thrombus as illustrated in Figure 1A. This local release enables it to bind rapidly to the fibrin where t-PA resists inactivation by its inhibitors. However, when t-PA is infused peripherally in pharmacological doses, interaction with inhibitors is unavoidable, as illustrated in Figure 1B. As a result, some of the infused t-PA is lost in complexes with inhibitors and important inhibitors are consumed. As a result, the natural defenses against the non-specific proteolytic effects of plasmin are thereby compromised.

These changes are an inevitable consequence of prolonged infusions of t-PA. It may be said that t-PA was not designed by nature to be infused, rather it is exceptionally well-suited for bolus injection because of its high fibrin affinity. By contrast, pro-UK is ill-suited for bolus therapy since it has little fibrin affinity, but is well-suited for prolonged systemic infusions because of its zymogenicity. These important differences in the physiological and pharmacological properties of t-PA and pro-UK are illustrated in Figures 1A and 1B. These differences may be usefully exploited clinically though these concepts remain to be evaluated in clinical trials.

For example, conditions in which more prolonged thrombolytic therapy is indicated, such as unstable angina, may be more safely treated with pro-UK since it can be administered in doses which are unlikely to impair hemostasis in contrast to t-PA. It has to be determined, however, whether pro-UK will be effective at such doses. On the other hand, the rapid induction of a thrombolytic state is probably better accomplished by t-PA, preferably by bolus injection. Pro-urokinase is relatively slow in its onset of action at lower doses and is converted to UK in the presence of plasminemia, thereby limiting therapy with high doses. The advantage of pro-UK over UK may be lost at doses at which a major non-specific effect is induced.

At fibrin-specific concentrations, clot lysis by pro-UK *in vitro* is preceded by a lag phase, whereas that by t-PA is not.[23] Although in certain animal species, the dose response curve of pro-UK may be more linear, as shown by Spriggs *et al.*,[24] early clinical trials in acute myocardial infarction showed a relatively slow reperfusion rate when relatively low, fibrin selective doses of pro-UK were used.[25]

This lag phase was attenuated and pro-UK-induced clot lysis potentiated when the clot was gently pretreated with plasmin.[21] Harpel *et al.*[26] have shown that plasmin exposes new plasminogen binding sites on fibrin. These new sites consist of carboxyterminal lysines, whereas on intact fibrin only internal lysine residues are available. Therefore, it appeared that pro-UK-induced fibrinolysis is dependent on the availability of carboxyterminal lysine-bound plasminogen.[23]

By contrast, fibrin-bound t-PA-induced clot lysis was shown not to be affected by plasmin-pretreament of a fibrin clot. It should be noted that a plasma milieu was found to be important for the demonstration of this effect since certain plasma inhibitors appear to be required to confine the proteolytic process to the fibrin surface. It was the fibrin-bound t-PA which was found preferentially to activate plasminogen bound to an internal lysine on fibrin. This was apparent from the finding that fibrinolysis by t-PA was not inhibited by carboxypeptidase-B (which removes C-terminal lysines) and was not potentiated by exposure of carboxyterminal lysines on fibrin. These complementary modes of action of t-PA and pro-UK were postulated to be the principal mechanism responsible for their synergy in fibrinolysis. They also explain the lag phase of pro-UK induced clot lysis and the more linear fibrinolytic effect of t-PA.[23]

From the foregoing, it follows that any plasminogen activator or any agent which releases t-PA from the vessel wall is apt to potentiate the thrombolytic properties of pro-UK. Thus, it has been shown that pro-UK-induced clot lysis *in vitro*[27] or in patients with acute myocardial infarction[28] is potentiated by a small, subtherapeutic bolus of UK. This is sufficient to initiate some clot lysis and thereby generate the new plasminogen binding sites on fibrin required by pro-UK. Similarly, a bolus of heparin has been found to potentiate the thrombolytic effect of pro-UK. Attempts to demonstrate an effect of heparin on pro-UK-induced clot lysis *in vitro* have been unsuccessful (unpublished observations) suggesting that this is an *in vivo* phenomenon. Since heparin has been shown by Fareed *et al.*[29] to release t-PA *in vivo*, we have postulated that it is the t-PA released from the endothelium which is responsible for the potentiation of pro-UK induced thrombolysis by heparin.

The differences in the properties of t-PA and pro-UK, summarized in Table 1, provide each activator with certain clinical indications for which it may be especially suitable. The ones for which pro-UK's properties may make it the activator of choice are summarized in Table 2. It should be noted, however, that this list is based on theoretical considerations only and remains to be verified by clinical trials. What has been shown is that in contrast to pro-UK, a prolonged (4–12 hours) infusion of t-PA, even at doses of only 0.5–2.5 miligrams per hour is associated with substantial fibrinogenolysis.[30] Moreover, a prolonged infusion of t-PA for the treatment of unstable angina[31] or pulmonary embolism[32] was associated with a relatively high incidence of bleeding.

Table 1 *Comparison of the thrombolytic properties of pro-UK and t-PA*

	pro-UK	*t-PA*
Fibrin specificity	+	+
Fibrin clot binding	?0	+
Zymogenicity in plasma	+	0
Suitable for prolonged infusions	+	0
Rapid onset of action	0/+	+

Table 2 *Clinical indications for which the zymogenic properties of pro-UK make it potentially the activator of choice*

1. Deep vein thrombosis and pulmonary embolism – in which the thrombus mass may necessitate prolonged (12–24 h) treatment.
2. Unstable angina – prolonged (days) treatment desirable and should be possible with pro-UK without inducing a hemorrhagic diathesis.
3. Transient ischemic attacks – (as above).
4. Prevention of rethrombosis following PTCA or after acute lytic therapy – use of relatively low-dose infusions for hours–days.

Monotherapy with t-PA or pro-UK

Extensive clinical trials involving several thousand patients with acute coronary thrombosis have been completed with t-PA which provide sufficient data for some conclusions. Unfortunately, the clinical experience with pro-UK is far more limited but certain tentative conclusions may nevertheless be ventured.

It is evident that unexpectedly high doses of t-PA are required for efficacy. Dose-ranging studies went up to 150 mg but because of the fear of intracranial hemorrhage, a dose limit of 100 mg is now recommended for the treatment of acute myocardial infarction. This dose requirement is in sharp and somewhat paradoxical contrast to the far lower dose requirements of the older, non-specific plasminogen activators, SK and UK. Moreover, the heralded and desirable fibrin-specificity of t-PA is all but lost at these doses. Although coronary patency rates appear to be somewhat higher with t-PA than with SK, especially when older thrombi are involved, the clinical importance of this difference remains to be established. The GISSI-2 trial in which mortality and morbidity associated with treatment with t-PA or SK are being compared should provide this information.

Similarly, at fibrin-selective doses, pro-UK is also relatively ineffective, inducing only a 51% reperfusion rate.[25] At high doses (80 mg), a patency rate of 72% was obtained in the PRIMI study[33] which is a patency rate comparable with that reported in most studies with t-PA. However, at this high dose of pro-UK extensive plasminemia occurred as reflected by an 80% reduction in fibrinogen. Since pro-UK is very sensitive to activation by plasmin, the PRIMI trial results may more acurately reflect the effects of high doses of UK, since most if not all the pro-UK was probably converted to UK. It is therefore quite possible that the same results would have been

Table 3 *Potential advantages of therapy with combinations of t-PA and pro-UK*

1. Superior efficacy – as a result of activation of all available fibrin-bound plasminogen and the preservation of the plasminogen reservoir in plasma.
2. Avoidance of systemic lytic state – little non-specific plasminogen activation.
3. Lower incidence of bleeding complications – the reserve of clotting factors and essential inhibitors important for hemostasis not compromised.
4. Improved myocardial salvage – tissue necrosis resulting from interstitial hemorrhage and the generation of anaphylotoxins is avoided.
5. Lower cost – less total amount of the activators needed due to their synergy.

obtained if UK rather than pro-UK had been used. Since pro-UK to UK conversion was not measured in the PRIMI study, this interpretation of the findings needs still to be evaluated.

These high dose-requirements of t-PA or pro-UK, when they are used alone to induce thrombolysis, can be explained by their respective mechanisms of plasminogen activation. As described above, at fibrin-selective doses t-PA and pro-UK each activates only a portion of the total fibrin-bound plasminogen. One selectively activates the internal lysine bound plasminogen and the other the carboxyterminal lysine bound plasminogen. Only at high non-specific doses will t-PA or pro-UK activate the alternate pool of fibrin-bound plasminogen. Efficacy is greatly improved at these high doses, but at the cost of specificity. Moreover, the economic cost of using large amounts of these expensive activators must be considered.

The fibrinolytic efficacy of combination therapy and the sequential effects of t-PA and pro-UK

The corollary of the above thesis is that only when t-PA and pro-UK are combined can effective coronary thrombolysis be achieved without sacrificing specificity. This has indeed been shown to be the case in both animal models[24] and in pilot clinical trials.[13, 34] Fractional combinations of t-PA and pro-UK corresponding to about 22%[34] and 72%[13] have been reported to give patency rates equivalent to those reported for monotherapy. Any fractional combination of less than 100% of monotherapy indicates that the two agents are synergistic according to the criteria established by Berenbaum.[35] These clinical studies, therefore, confirm the finding of synergy demonstrated previously in clot lysis studies with combinations of t-PA and pro-UK *in vitro*.[21, 23] Pilot clinical trials of synergistic combinations are continuing in order to establish the optimal combination of t-PA and pro-UK and then to compare this combination with the results of monotherapy.

The potential advantages of combination therapy are three-fold. First, by avoiding a systemic lytic effect, the toxic effects of plasmin (recently reviewed[36]) may be prevented. Second, specificity permits conservation of the plasminogen reservoir in plasma shown originally by Chesterman *et al.*[37] to be important for optimal fibrinolysis. Third, the lower dose requirements should reduce the cost of the treatment. All of these potential advantages which are listed in Table 3 remain to be established by clinical trials.

As noted above, t-PA and pro-UK have different and complementary mechanisms for activating fibrin-bound plasminogen, and their disparate effects had been invoked to explain their synergy.[23] In addition, t-PA and pro-UK are also sequential in their fibrinolytic effects, as recently reviewed.[11] Tissue plasminogen activator initiates clot lysis by binding to its receptor sequence on fibrin and forming a ternary complex with plasminogen as demonstrated by Hoylaerts *et al.*[38] The plasminogen involved in this ternary complex is bound to an internal lysine[23] believed to be the internal lysine residue Aα-Lys-157 according to Niewenhuizen *et al.*[39, 40] This residue is present on intact fibrin. Naturally occurring clot lysis is probably initiated when t-PA is released from the vessel wall near the site of a thrombus (Fig. 1A) and this physiological design for fibrinolysis can be better replicated pharmacologically by a bolus of t-PA rather than by an infusion.

After lysis has been initiated, plasminogen from the plasma binds to new binding sites on the fibrin clot, the carboxyterminal lysines created by plasmin cleavage of the intact α, β and γ chains of fibrin. Only at this point can pro-UK participate in the fibrinolytic process by activating the carboxyterminal lysine bound plasminogen on fibrin.[23] In the process, pro-UK is activated, thereby considerably amplifying local plasminogen activation.

The activation of pro-UK represents an important element in pro-UK induced fibrinolysis.

Pro-urokinase is a zymogen with a low intrinsic fibrinolytic activity and activation to UK has been shown to be associated with a 250-fold increase in plasminogen-activating activity.[41, 42] Both plasmin[18] and kallikrein[43] activate pro-UK by hydrolysing the Lys-158–Ile-159 peptide bond.[44] The activation by plasmin provides a positive feedback through the generation of UK which accelerates plasmin formation on the fibrin surface and was originally postulated to be a cardinal feature of pro-UK induced clot lysis.[45]

In one study of the kinetics of plasminogen activation by pro-UK, Collen *et al.*[46] concluded that pro-UK had a catalytic efficiency slightly greater even than that of UK. Its designation as a proenzyme was consequently challenged. Moreover, in a study measuring pro-UK activation during clot lysis *in vitro*, it was found that lysis was associated with only ≈10% conversion of pro-UK to UK.[17] These findings suggested that pro-UK itself might be responsible for fibrinolysis and that activation to UK was incidental and perhaps irrelevant.

This possibility was recently evaluated with two plasmin-resistant mutants of pro-UK. These non-activatable forms of pro-UK were found to have only about 1% of the clot lysing effect of native pro-UK, indicating that pro-UK activation was important for fibrinolysis. Their fibrinolytic activity was, however, potentiated by t-PA with which both mutants were shown to be synergistic.[47] It was concluded that pro-UK activation is importantly involved in pro-UK induced clot lysis, as also confirmed by a recent study by Lijnen *et al.*[48] The synergy with t-PA in fibrinolysis appears to be a function of pro-UK itself rather than an accelerated activation to UK by the effects of t-PA.[47]

The molecular mechanism by which pro-UK is activated to UK is not known. On the clot surface, it is likely that fibrin bound plasmin is responsible, but whether it is the internal lysine bound plasmin generated by t-PA or a carboxyterminal lysine bound plasmin generated by the intrinsic activity of pro-UK remains to be determined. Alternatively, kallikrein has also been implicated by Ichinose *et al.*[43] as a physiological activator of pro-UK, and may be involved under certain conditions. After all, ever since the demise of John Hageman due to massive pulmonary embolism,[49] suspicion has been drawn to a relationship between the contact activation pathway and fibrinolysis. Since kallikrein is a relatively weak plasminogen activator, its fibrinolytic effect is believed to be mediated through the activation of a plasma pro-activator thought to be pro-UK. Whatever the precise mechanism turns out to be, the activation of pro-UK to UK appears to be a critical step in pro-UK induced fibrinolysis.

The sequential relationship between t-PA and pro-UK in fibrinolysis has also been found *in vivo* in experimental animals. Sequential doses of t-PA followed by pro-UK were shown by Collen *et al.* to be synergistic in their lysis of jugular vein thrombi. By contrast, when the sequence was reversed and pro-UK was given first, relatively poor clot lysis and no synergy was found.[50]

The optimal combination of t-PA and pro-UK for therapeutic thrombolysis has not been determined, but all evidence from *in vitro* and experimental animal studies suggests that t-PA should be used to initiate therapy. One approach would be to replicate the natural design for fibrinolysis, that is to give a bolus (or boluses) of t-PA followed by an infusion of pro-UK. This approach takes advantage of the differences in properties of the activators. The follow-up pro-UK infusion, if prolonged, possibly at a lower dose, may also help to prevent rethrombosis. The administration of pro-UK would, of course, be much simplified if a modification to prolong its half-life, which is only 5–8 minutes, were to be developed. Such a modification of pro-UK appears eminently rational whereas this is not necessarily the case for t-PA since a longer half-life would be associated with a greater non-specific proteolytic effect. A proposal for a protocol for combination therapy based on available limited clinical data, as well as on theoretical considerations, is provided in Table 4.

UK and pro-UK

The main difference between UK and pro-UK is in their enzymatic activities, the catalytic activity of the latter being no more than about 0.4% of the former against either plasminogen or synthetic substrate.[41] This difference in activities is related to a conformational change. Hydrodynamic studies by Barlow *et al.*[51] have indicated that pro-UK is a more compact molecule as reflected by its sedimentation coefficient. An important function of the pro-UK form can be said to be that of transport. Thus, it enables UK to reach a clot intact without disturbing hemostasis.

Table 4 *Outline of a proposed clinical protocol for coronary thrombolysis with a combination of t-PA and pro-UK*

Objective: 80–90% patency rate with little or no non-specific effect (as reflected by fibrinogen degradation) and little or no rethrombosis.

1. Give 160 mg aspirin p.o.
2. Administer an i.v. bolus of 5 mg t-PA to initiate lysis as soon as diagnosis is suspected.
3. Promptly start infusion of pro-UK at rate of 20 mg per hour.
4. After 10 min, give second bolus of 5 mg t-PA.
5. At 20 min, give third bolus of 5 mg t-PA.
6. At 60 min, reduce pro-UK infusion rate to 10 mg per hour and continue for an additional 3 hours to lyse residual fibrin and to prevent rethrombosis.
7. At the end of pro-UK infusion, start i.v. heparin.

This protocol is based on the preliminary results of pilot trials and on the theoretical grounds reviewed.

That being the case, clinical indications for thrombolytic therapy in which the activator is delivered to the clot via a catheter, are probably better suited to the use of UK than pro-UK. For example, intra-arterial fibrinolytic therapy with UK has been used successfully in peripheral arterial occlusions.[52] For this indication, UK appears to be superior to SK, perhaps because with the latter a portion of the plasminogen is taken up in the activator complex and therefore is unavailable for lysis. There is no obvious rationale for delivering pro-UK to a clot via a catheter since this would appear to be superfluous, and therefore, this is one clinical example of an indication where UK may be the thrombolytic agent of choice.

Pro-urokinase is the latent form of UK and is therefore better suited for clinical settings in which this zymogenic property can be effectively utilized, as in systemic intravenous infusions for acute thrombolysis or more long term subacute thrombolysis or even for prevention. The latter would become practical only with a modification to give pro-UK a long half-life and may mimic its physiological role. Pro-urokinase is available normally in the blood plasma reservoir but its importance in fibrinolysis has not been established.[53, 54] This is in part due to the inactivation of pro-UK by thrombin which has confounded some *in vitro* studies.[55] Moreover, pro-UK is incompletely precipitated in the euglobulin fraction, commonly used to measure fibrinolytic activity, further complicating assessment of its physiological function. Nevertheless, its complementary properties and complementary mechanism of action compared with t-PA suggest that both activators are required for the normal defense against intravascular thrombosis.

Since pro-UK has little fibrinolytic activity against an intact clot, but is effective against slightly degraded clots, UK can be substituted pharmacologically for t-PA in combination with pro-UK.[27] However, this combination is apt to be less effective since the fibrinolytic effect of a bolus of UK is transient whereas that of t-PA is more sustained due to its fibrin affinity. Nevertheless, an initial bolus of UK has been shown to potentiate pro-UK-induced fibrinolysis.[28, 56] Compared with pro-UK monotherapy, the evidence suggests that a subtherapeutic dose of UK improves the efficiency of pro-UK and allows the dose to be reduced perhaps by as much as 50%. Moreover, the UK/pro-UK combination appears to be associated with less fibrinogen degradation than pro-UK alone for an equivalent patency rate. Since effective thrombolysis with pro-UK alone requires doses at which a significant conversion to UK undoubtedly occurs anyway, it may be more rational as well as more efficient to initiate lysis with a bolus of UK.

Summary and conclusions

The distinctive fibrinolytic properties of pro-UK are reviewed and contrasted to those of t-PA. An important difference between the activators is the zymogenicity of pro-UK which makes it possible to administer a prolonged infusion without compromising hemostasis or triggering the other biochemical events associated with non-specific plasminogen activation. On the other hand, when used as monotherapy, high doses of pro-UK are required at which plasminemia occurs with the consequent systemic activation of pro-UK to UK. The advantage of pro-UK over UK may thereby be lost. This problem can be avoided by using lower doses of pro-UK. However, these are optimally effective only if preceded by a bolus of UK or t-PA. The latter is preferred because of the synergy of t-PA and pro-UK in fibrinolysis, related to their sequential and complementary mechanisms of action.

Proposals are offered for clinical applications of monotherapy with pro-UK and combination therapy with t-PA or UK, based on their known mechanisms of action and on clinical trial data.

References

1. Gurewich V, Lipinska I, Lipinski B, Exercise-induced fibrinolytic activity and its effect on the degradation of fibrinogen, fibrin and fibrin-like precipitates. *Thrombos. Res. 5*, 1974, 647–656.
2. Lipinski V, Nowak A, Gurewich V, Fibrinolysis versus fibrinogenolysis in man: Resistance of fibrinogen to breakdown by fibrinolytic activity induced by venous occlusion. *Experientia 30*, 1974, 84–85.
3. Gurewich V, Nowak A, Lipinska I, Lipinski B, The resistance of soluble derivatives of fibrinogen and the sensitivity of its insoluble forms to fibrinolytic degradation in blood. *Thrombos. Diathes. Haemorrh. 32*, 1974, 582–591.
4. Marder V J, Shulman W R, High molecular weight derivatives of human fibrinogen produced by plasmin. II. Mechanism of their anticoagulant activity. *J. Biol. Chem. 244*, 1969, 2120–2124.
5. Sueishi K, Nanno D, Tanaka K, Permeability enhancing and chemotactic activities of lower molecular weight degradation products. *Thrombos. Haemostas. 45*, 1981, 90–94.
6. Waller B F, Rothbaum D A, Pinkerton C A, Cowley M J, Linnemeier T J, Orr C, Irons M, Helmuth R A, Wills E R, Anst C, Status of myocardium and infarct-related coronary artery in 19 necropsy patients with acute recanalization using pharmacologic (streptokinase, r-tissue plasminogen activator) or combined types of reperfusion therapy. *J. Am. Coll. Cardiol. 9*, 1987, 785–801.
7. Niewiarowski S, Senyi A F, Gillies P, Plasmin-induced platelet aggregation and platelet release reaction. Effects on hemostasis. *J. Clin. Invest., 52*, 1973, 1647–1659.
8. Godal H C, Hale I, Studies of the clot promoting effect of large concentrations of streptokinase. *Scand. J. Clin. Lab. 15*, 1963, 375–379.

9. Hirsh J, Buchanan M, Glynn M F, Mustard J F, Effect of activation of the fibrinolytic mechanism on experimental platelet rich thrombi in rabbits. *J. Lab. Clin. Med. 72*, 1968, 245–255.
10. Bennett W R, Yawn D H, Migliove P J, Young J B, Pratt C M, Raizner A E, Roberts R, Bolli R, Activation of the complement system by recombinant tissue plasminogen activator. *J. Am. Coll. Cardiol. 10*, 1987, 627–633.
11. Gurewich V, The sequential, complementary and synergistic activation of fibrin-bound plasminogen by tissue plasminogen activator and pro-urokinase. *Fibrinolysis 3*, 1989, 59–66.
12. Collen D, Stassen J M, Stump D C, Verstraete M, *In vivo* synergism of thrombolytic agents. *Circulation 74*, 1986, 838–842.
13. Bode C, Shoenermark S, Schaler S, Banman H, Richardt G, Dietz R, Gurewich V, Kubler W, Intravenous thrombolytic therapy with a combination single-chain urokinase-type plasminogen activator and recombinant tissue-type plasminogen activator in acute myocardial infarction. *Clinical Res. 37(2)*, 1989, 247A.
14. Marder V, Pharmacology of thrombolytic agents. Implications for therapy of coronary artery thrombosis. *Circulation 68*, 1983, I-2 – I-5.
15. Husain S S, Gurewich V, Lipinski B, Purification of a new high MW single chain form of urokinase (UK) from urine. *Thrombo. Haemost. 47*, 1981, 11 (Abst.).
16. Husain S S, Gurewich V, Purification and partial characterization of a single chain, high molecular weight form of urokinase from human urine. *Arch. Biochem. Biophy. 220(1)*, 1983, 31–38.
17. Pannell R, Gurewich V, Pro-urokinase – a study of its stability in plasma and a mechanism for its selective fibrinolytic effect. *Blood 67*, 1986, 1215–1223.
18. Gurewich V, Pannell R, Louie S, Kelley P, Suddith R L, Greenlee R, Effective and fibrin-specific clot lysis by a zymogen precursor form of urokinase (pro-urokinase). A study *in vitro* and in two animal species. *J. Clin. Invest. 73*, 1984, 1731–1739.
19. Van de Werf F, Nobuhara M, Collen D, Coronary thrombolysis with human single chain urokinase-type plasminogen activator (pro-urokinase) in patients with acute myocardial infarction. *Ann. Int. Med. 104*, 1986, 345–348.
20. Lijnen H R, Zammarron C, Blaber M, Winkler M E, Collen D, Activation of plasminogen by pro-urokinase. I Mechanism. *J. Biol. Chem. 261*, 1986, 1253–1258.
21. Gurewich V, Pannell R, A comparative study of the efficacy and specificity of tissue plasminogen activator and pro-urokinase: demonstration of synergism and of different thresholds of non-selectivity. *Thromb. Res. 44*, 1986, 217–228.
22. Heckman C M, Loskutoff D J, Kinetic analysis of the interactions between plasminogen activator inhibitor I and both urokinase and tissue plasminogen activator. *Arch. Biochem. Biophys. 262*, 199–210.
23. Pannell R, Black J, Gurewich V, The complementary modes of action of tissue plasminogen activator (t-PA) and pro-urokinase (pro-UK) by which their synergistic effect on clot lysis may be explained. *J. Clin. Invest. 81*, 1988, 853–859.
24. Spriggs D J, Stassen J M, Hashimoto Y, Collen D, Thrombolytic properties of human tissue-type plasminogen activator, single chain urokinase-type plasminogen activator, and synergistic combinations in venous thrombosis models in dogs and rabbits. *Blood 73*, 1989, 1207–1212.
25. Loscalzo J, Wharton T P, Kirshenbaum J M, Levine H J, Flaherty J T, Topol E J, Ramaswamy K, Kosowsky B D, Salem D N, Ganz P, Brinker J A, Gurewich V, Muller J E, and the Prourokinase for Myocardial Infarction Study Group: Clot Selective Coronary Thrombolysis with Prourokinase. *Circulation 79(4)*, 1989, 776–782.

26. Harpel P C, Chang T S, Verderber E, Tissue plasminogen activator and urokinase mediate the binding of Glu-plasminogen to plasma fibrin I: Evidence for new binding sites in plasmin-degraded fibrin I. *J. Biol. Chem. 260*, 1985, 4432–4440.
27. Gurewich V, Experiences with pro-urokinase and potentiation of its fibrinolytic effect by urokinase and by tissue plasminogen activator. *J. Am. Coll. Cardiol. 10(5)*, 1987, 16B–21B.
28. Bode C, Schoenermark S, Schuller G, Zimmerman R, Schwarz F, Kuebler W, Efficacy of intravenous prourokinase and a combination of prourokinase and urokinase in acute myocardial infarction. *Am. J. Cardiol. 61*, 1988, 971–974.
29. Fareed J, Walenga J, Hoppensteadt D, Messmore H L, Studies on the pro-fibrinolytic action of heparin and its fractions. *Semin. Thrombos. Haemostas. 11(2)*, 1985, 199–207.
30. Earnshaw J J, Westby J C, Gregson R H S, Makin G S, Hopkinson B R, Local thrombolytic therapy for acute peripheral arterial ischaemia with tissue plasminogen activator: a dose ranging study. *Brit. J. Surg. 75*, 1988, 1196–1200.
31. Gold H K, Johns J A, Lenbach R C, *et al*, A randomized blind, placebo-controlled study of recombinant tissue plasminogen activator in patients with unstable angina pectoris. *Circulation 75*, 1987, 1192–1199.
32. Goldhaber S Z, Kessler C M, Heit J *et al*, Randomized controlled clinical trial of recombinant tissue plasminogen activator versus urokinase in the treatment of acute pulmonary embolism. *Lancet 1*, 1988, 293–298.
33. PRIMI Trial Study Group: Randomized double blind trial of recombinant pro-urokinase against streptokinase in acute myocardial infarction. *Lancet 1*, 1989, 863–867.
34. Collen D, Van de Werf F, Coronary arterial thrombolysis with low dose synergistic combinations of recombinant tissue type plasminogen activator and recombinant single chain urokinase type plasminogen activator for acute myocardial infarction. *Am. J. Cardiol. 60*, 1987, 431–434.
35. Berenbaum M C, Synergy, additivism and antagonism in immunosuppression. A critical review. *Clin. Exp. Immunol. 28*, 1977, 1–18.
36. Gurewich V, The importance of fibrin specificity in therapeutic thrombolysis and the rationale of using sequential and synergistic combinations of t-PA and pro-urokinase. *Semin. Thrombos. Haemostas. 15(2)*, 1989, 123–128.
37. Chesterman C N, Allington M J, Sharp A A, Relationship of Plasminogen activator to fibrin. *Nature 238*, 1972, 15–17.
38. Hoylaerts M, Rijken D C, Lijnen H R, Collen D, Kinetics of the activation of plasminogen by human tissue plasminogen activator. Role of fibrin. *J. Biol. Chem. 257*, 1982, 2912–2919.
39. Nieuwenhuizen W, Vermond A, Voskuilen M, Traas D W, Verheijen J H, Identification of a site in fibrin(ogen) which is involved in the acceleration of plasminogen activation by tissue-type plasminogen activator. *Biochim. Biophys. Acta 748*, 1983, 86–92.
40. Nieuwenhuizen W, Voskuilen M, Vermond A, Veeneman G, Boom J V, Lysine residue A-α157 of fibrinogen plays a crucial role in the acceleration of the plasminogen activation by tissue plasminogen activator (t-PA). *Fibrinolysis*, 1986, Abstract 9.
41. Pannell R and Gurewich V, The activation of plasminogen by single-chain urokinase or by two-chain urokinase – A demonstration that single chain urokinase has a low catalytic activity (pro-urokinase). *Blood 69*, 1987, 22–26.
42. Petersen L C, Lund L R, Dano K, Nielsen L S, Skriver L, One-chain urokinase type plasminogen activator from human sarcoma cells is a proenzyme with little or no intrinsic activity. *J. Biol. Chem. 263*, 1988, 11189–11195.
43. Ichinose A, Fujikawa K, Suyama T, The activation of pro-urokinase by plasma kallikrein and its inactivation by thrombin. *J. Biol. Chem. 261*, 1986, 3486–3489.

44. Gunzler W A, Steffens G J, Otting F, Buse G, Flohe L, Structural relationship between high and low molecular mass urokinases. *Hoppe-Seyler's Z. Physiol. Chem. 363*, 1982, 133–141.
45. Gurewich V, Characterization and thrombolytic properties of pro-urokinase. In *Thrombolysis: Biological and Therapeutic Properties of New Thrombolytic Agents*, Verstraete M and Collen D (eds), Churchill Livingstone, 1985, pp. 92–110.
46. Collen D, Zamarron C, Lijnen H R, Hoylaerts M, Activation of plasminogen by pro-urokinase. II. Kinetics. *J. Biol. Chem. 261*, 1986, 1259–1266.
47. Gurewich V, Pannell R, Broeze R J, Mao J-I, Characterization of the intrinsic fibrinolytic properties of pro-urokinase through a study of plasmin resistant mutant forms produced by site specific mutagenesis of lysine-158. *J. Clin. Invest. 82*, 198, 1956–1962.
48. Lijnen H R, Van Hoef B, De Cock F, Collen D, The mechanism of plasminogen activation and fibrin dissolution by single chain urokinase type plasminogen activator in a plasma milieu *in vitro*. *Blood 73*, 1989, 1864–1877.
49. Ratnoff O D, Busse R J, Sheon R P, The demise of John Hageman. *N. Engl. J. Med. 279*, 1968, 760–761.
50. Collen D, Stassen J M, DeCock F, Synergistic effect on thrombolysis of sequential infusion of tissue type plasminogen activator (t-PA), single chain urokinase-type plasminogen activator (scu-PA), and urokinase in the rabbit jugular vein thrombosis model. *Thrombos. Haemostas. 58*, 1987, 943–946.
51. Barlow G, Firestone S L, Gurewich V, Hydrodynamic and biophysical studies on single chain and two-chain urokinase. *Biophys. J. 51*, 1987, 13a.
52. Belkin M, Belkin B, Bucknam C A, Straub J, Lowe R, Intra-arterial fibrinolytic therapy. *Arch. Surg. 121*, 1986, 769–772.
53. Wun T-C, Capuano A, Spontaneous fibrinolysis in whole plasma. Identification of tissue activator related protein as the major plasminogen activator causing spontaneous activity *in vitro*. *J. Biol. Chem. 260*, 5061–5066.
54. Gurewich V, Emmons F and Pannell R, Spontaneous clot lysis in whole human plasma by endogenous tissue type and urokinase type plasminogen activators: demonstration of a promoting effect by t-PA and by platelets on urokinase. *Fibrinolysis 2*, 1988, 143–149.
55. Gurewich V, Pannell R, Inactivation of single chain urokinase (pro-urokinase) by thrombin and thrombin-like enzymes: Relevance of the finding to the interpretation of fibrin binding experiments. *Blood 69*, 1987, 769–772.
56. Kasper W, Meinertz T, Hohnloser S, Engler H, Hasler C, Rossler W, Wolfe H, Welzel D, Just H, Gurewich V, Coronary thrombolysis in man with prourokinase: improved efficacy with low dose urokinase. *Klin. Wochenschr. 66*, 1988, 109–114.

Chapter 8

PRE-HOSPITAL THROMBOLYSIS: A CHALLENGE?

Jean-Pierre Boissel

Claude Bernard University, Lyon, France and

Alain Leizorovicz

Unité de Pharmacologie Clinique, Lyon, France

Introduction

Since the first administration of streptokinase to patients developing a myocardial infarction (MI) by Fletcher in 1958, numerous clinical trials have been carried out to prove the efficacy of thrombolysis in acute MI. The cumulated evidence has demonstrated beyond any doubt that such treatment is beneficial and with low risk. Thrombolysis in acute myocardial infarction (AMI) might be the most precisely assessed of all medical procedures. Among the enormous bulk of data, indirect as well as more direct evidence suggests that the mortality risk reduction from thrombolysis decreases with the delay between onset of symptoms and administration of a thrombolytic agent. We will first review this evidence; then we will outline what the consequences of the hypothesis of decreasing benefit might be.

The onset of symptoms is viewed as the landmark for the beginning of the process. Although this is certainly not true, it is obvious there is no more relevant alternative. The delay from onset of symptoms to treatment (DOT) will be central in this paper.

Conceptual framework

Animal experiments

For decades animal models of AMI mainly in dogs and rats have been used to investigate pathophysiology of human AMI and drug effects. They are all based on the reduction of either coronary blood flow or oxygen supply to the myocardium. Before the cells are irreversibly injured restoration of blood flow or oxygen supply allows a partial or total recovery of heart function. The size of the experimental infarct is related to the duration of occlusion until reperfusion[1] (Fig. 1). Hence, in these animal models, time is an important component of the experimental process.

Pathology

Contributions of pathology to our present understanding of the time factor in AMI are summarized in a comprehensive model of myocardial ischemic states.[2,3] This model is shown in Figure 2. It integrates three dimensions, the last two being on the domain of pathology:

1. Time (none of the events except sudden death are instantaneous);
2. Stepwise coronary events: plaque ulceration, platelet aggregates, platelet thrombi and emboli, mural thrombus, occlusive thrombus;
3. Progressive myocardial involvement from sub-endocardium to epicardium, from reversible ischemia to infarction, from small size multifocal affected areas to massive lesion.

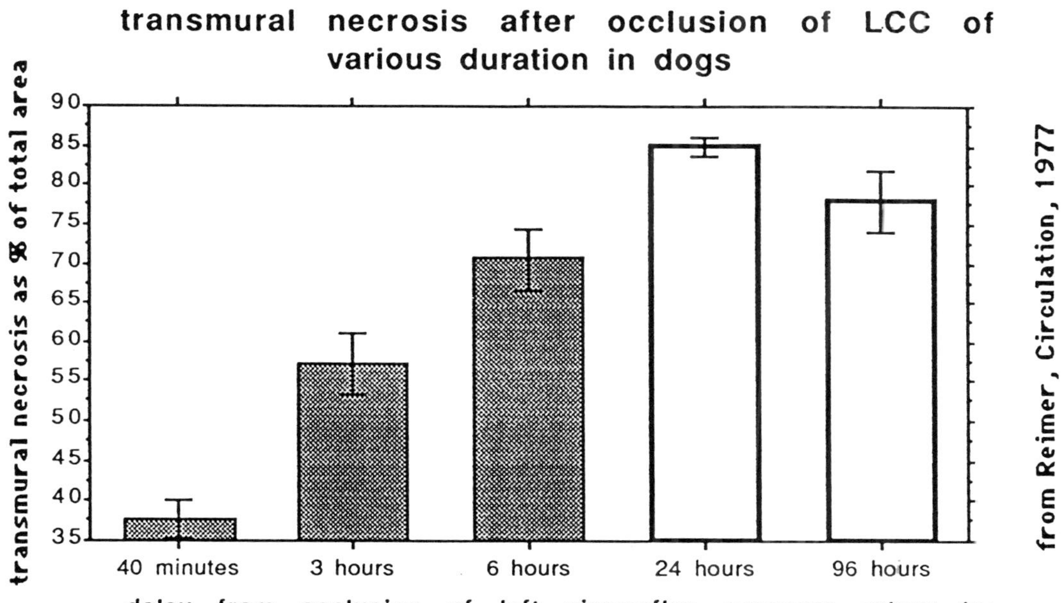

Figure 1 *Groups of dogs with left circumflex coronary artery ligation were reperfused for 2–4 days at 40 minutes (n=23), 3 hours (n=8), and 6 hours (n=8) after occlusion; others (open bars) had permanent occlusion for 24 hours (n=16) and 96 hours (n=3). From Reimer et al.*[1]

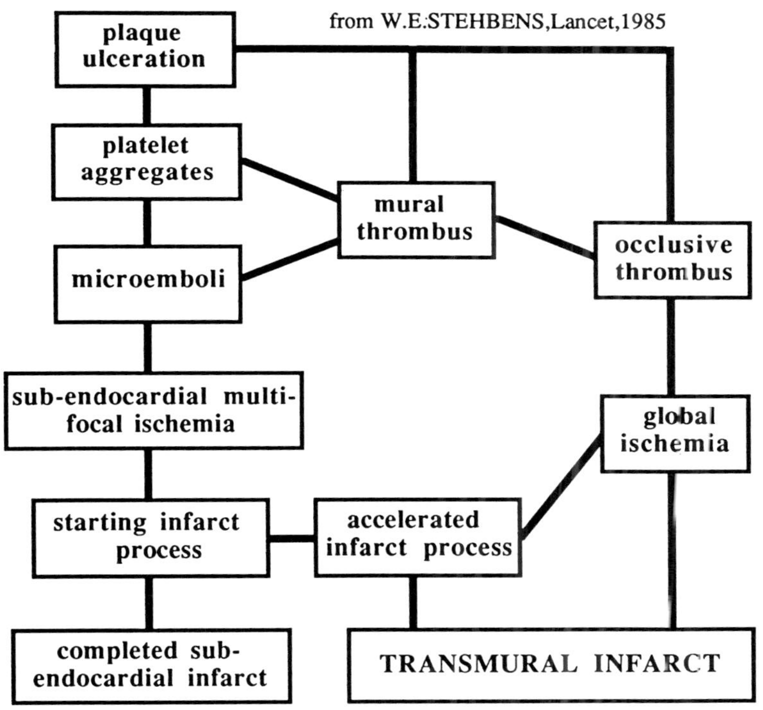

Figure 2 *This model of the mechanism of transmural infarction integrates findings from animal experiments and human pathology observations; it has been drawn on the basis of an editorial by Stehbens,* [3] *and a workshop.*[2]

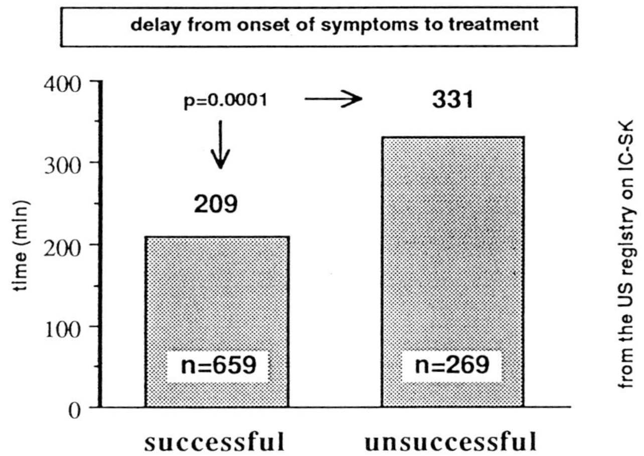

Figure 3 *Comparison of mean DOTs in successful and unsuccessful intracoronary streptokinase administration in the registry of the Society for Cardiac Angiography. From Kennedy et al.*[4]

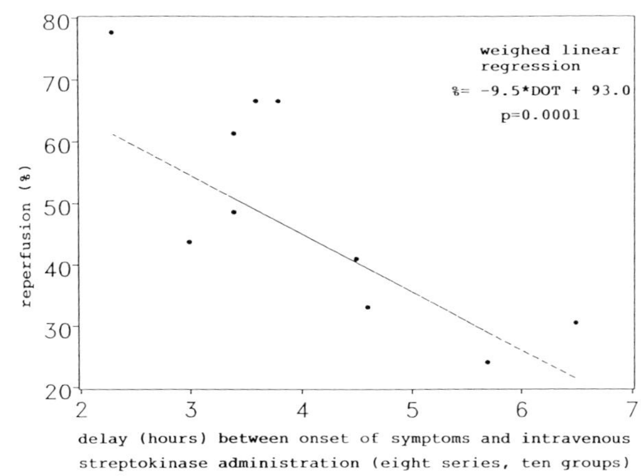

Figure 4 *Percentage of infarct-related arteries reperfused after intravenous streptokinase against DOT; data from table 1; the linear regression is weighed by the number of patients of each series.*

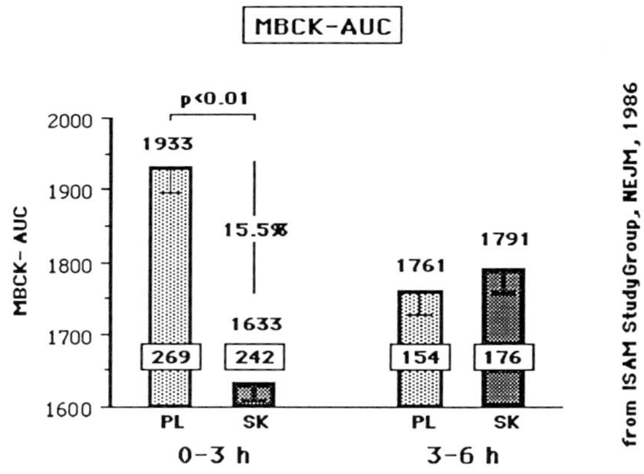

Figure 5 *Differences between streptokinase and placebo groups in terms of infarct size assessed by area under curve (AUC) of plasma MBCK concentration against time curve in patients treated within 3 hours or later. Figures in the rectangles are number of patients. From ISAM.*[13]

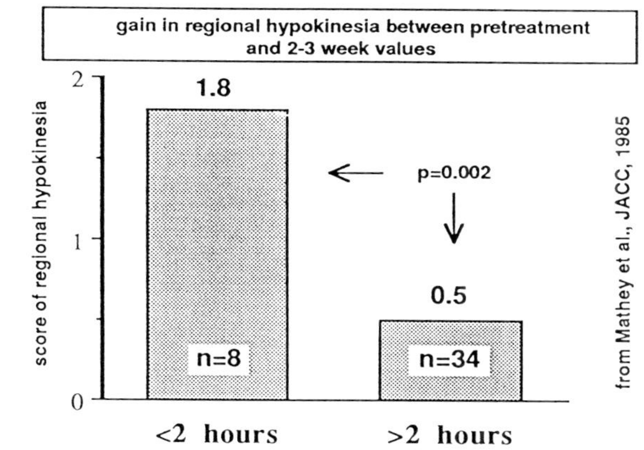

Figure 6 *Differences between gains over pre-treatment left ventricular regional hypokinesia score 2–3 weeks after treatment in patients treated within 2 hours and patients treated later. From Mathey et al.*[15]

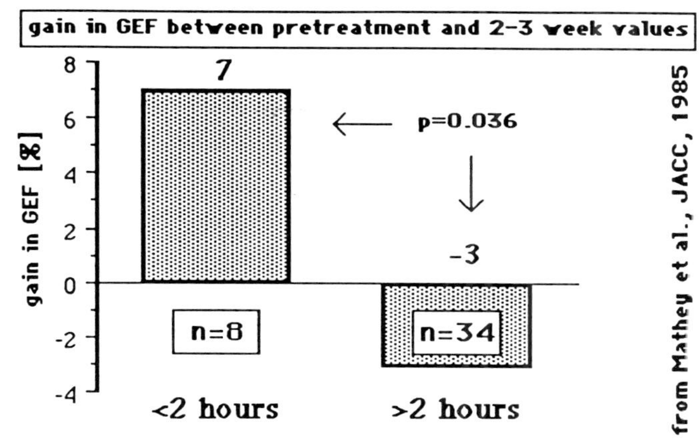

Figure 7 *Differences between gains over pre-treatment global left ventricular ejection fraction 2–3 weeks after treatment in patients within 2 hours and patients treated later. From Mathey et al.*[15]

Although this is purely speculative, sudden death which is not accounted for in this model and does not lead to histologic signs of infarction, can result from transient ischemia localized to few myocardial cells, caused by a platelet embolus.

Time could have another input in this model: there is some evidence that, as observed in unstable angina, the clot is not fixed but is continually built up and destroyed.

Acute myocardial infarction, a four dimension event

A doctor caring for a patient who develops a myocardial infarction, has to consider four disparate facets:

1. The underlying pathophysiological time-related process, a model of which has been proposed above;
2. Signs and symptoms i.e. the basis of diagnosis; definite diagnosis of myocardial infarction requires Q-waves and enzyme release; however Q-waves and enzyme release may not appear if the process is abated.

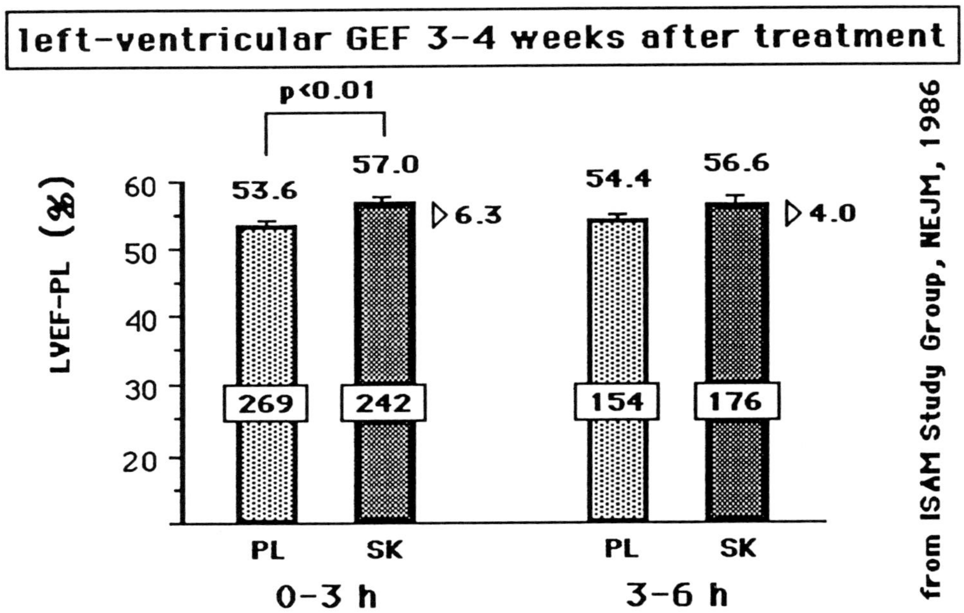

Figure 8 *Differences between streptokinase and placebo groups in global left ventricular ejection fraction in patients treated within 3 hours or later. Figures in the rectangles are number of patients. From ISAM.*[13]

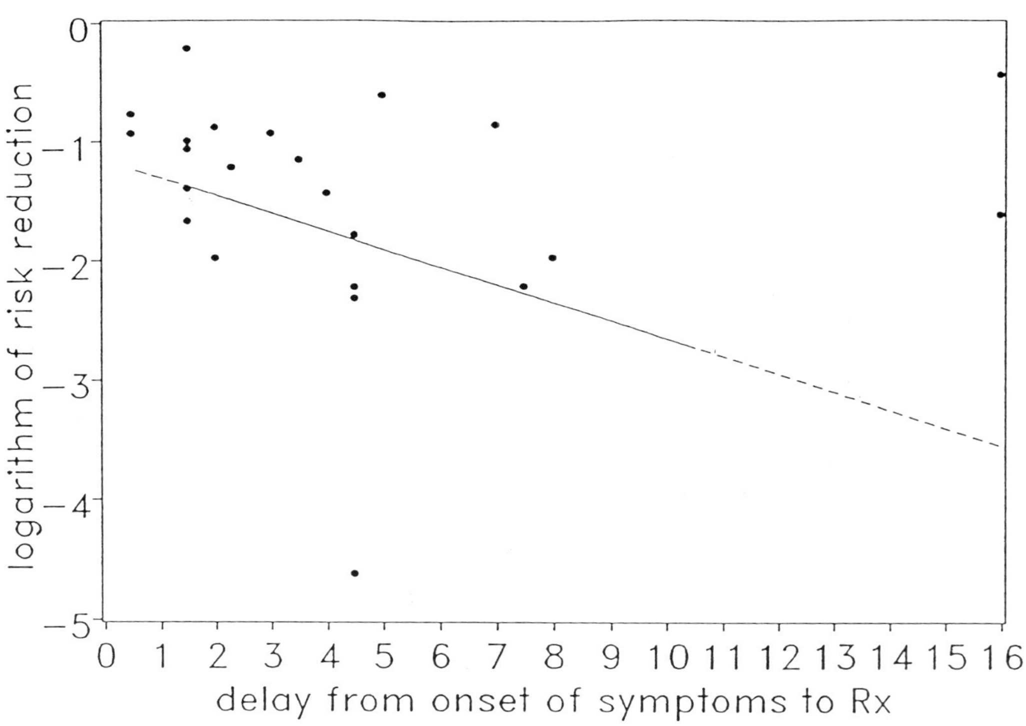

Figure 9 *Linear regression of the logarithm of risk reduction against the delay from onset of symptoms to treatment weighed by number of patients (p=0.0001); data from Table 2.*

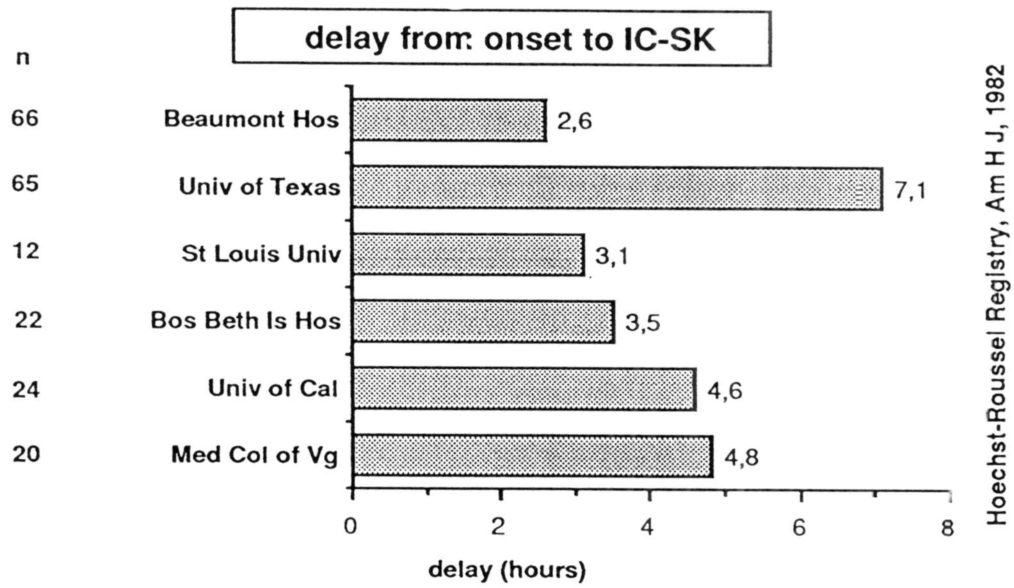

Figure 10 *Mean delays from onset of symptoms to intracoronary administration of streptokinase.*[23] *Intracoronary administration adds 30–60 minutes extra-delay over intravenous route.*

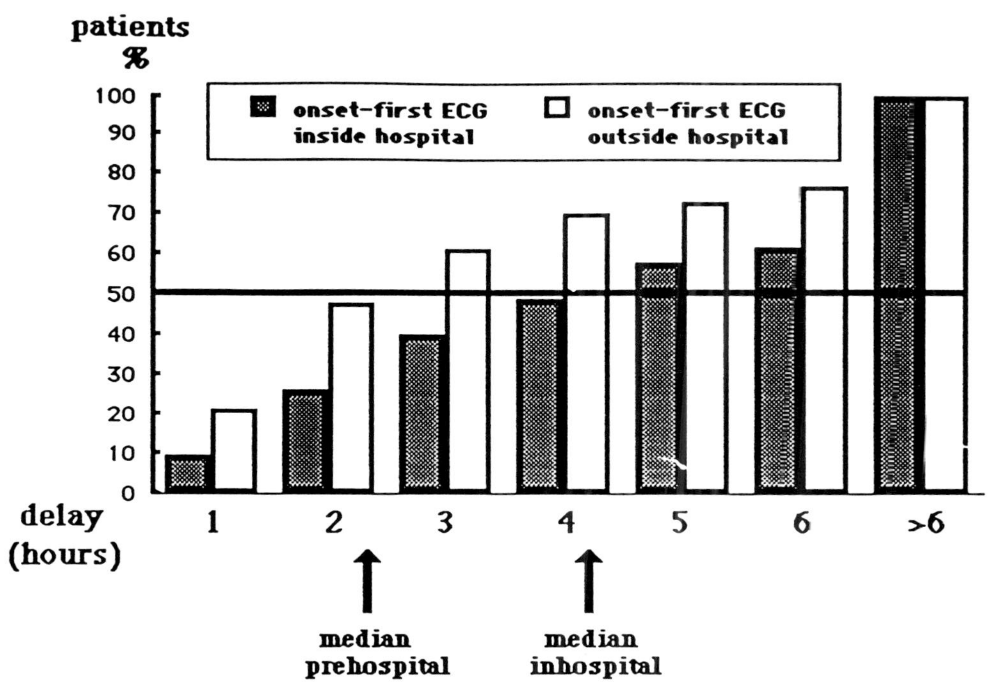

Figure 11 *Cumulative frequencies for delay between onset of symptoms and first ECG, outside versus inside hospital. Data from a prospective survey in eight European Cities.*[24]

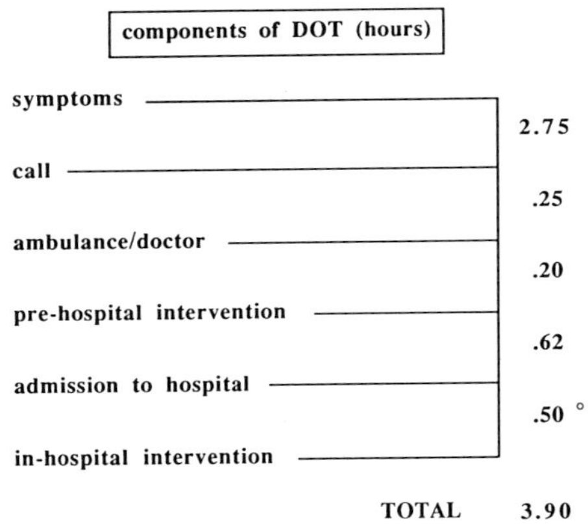

Figure 12 *Components of the delay from onset of symptoms to treatment. Figures up to admission were observed from median delays from onset of symptoms observed in MEXAP.*[29] *The time between admission and in-hospital intervention was reported by Herve et al.*[25,26]

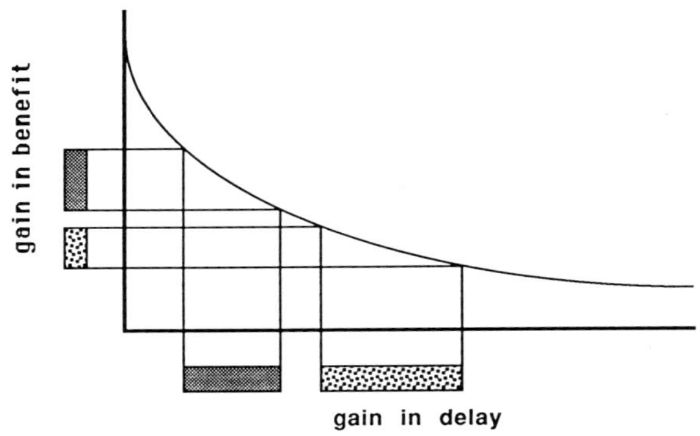

Figure 13 *Since the relationship benefit–DOT is likely to be exponential with a negative coefficient (see Figure 10, and equation (2),) a smaller and earlier reduction of DOT may lead to a greater increase in mortality risk reduction. Y-axis=benefit; X-axis=gain in delay.*

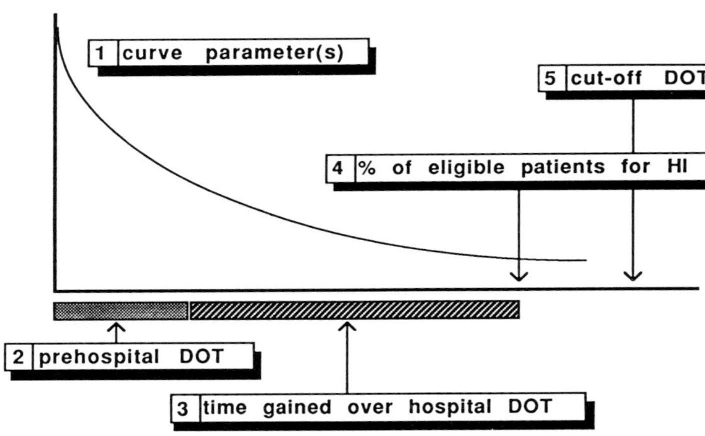

Figure 14 *The five components of the gain in benefit with earlier intervention. See text. Y-axis=benefit; X-axis=delay from onset of symptoms to intervention. HI: hospital intervention.*

3. The death hazard (mostly by ventricular arrythmia or cardiogenic shock), which could occur at any time before the process is completed.
4. The impairment of late survival because of progressive myocardium damage by the process.

Indirect observational evidence

It has been observed several times that patients with successful reopening are seen earlier than those whose infarct related artery remains occluded despite thrombolytic treatment. In the largest multicenter series with such data, the mean DOT for successful intracoronary thrombolysis was 3.5 hours as compared to 5.5 hours for unsuccessful treatment ($p = 0.0001$; Fig. 3[4]). This consistent observation suggests that older clots are more resistant to thrombolysis. An analysis of intravenous streptokinase reperfusion series (Table 1) shows a significant linear correlation between DOT and reperfusion rate, when only TIMI-grade 0.1 infarct related arteries at baseline are considered. This is shown in Figure 4. The weighed regression line has been obtained by pooling published data[5–12]:

$$\text{reperfusion rate } (\%) = -9.5 \times \text{DOT} + 83.0 \; (p = 0.0001) \qquad (1)$$

In a randomized study comparing 20, 50 and 100 mg of rtPA perfused over 90 min. McNeill *et al.* observed that in patients treated within 120 min (DOT), the patency rate was 81% (21/26), as compared to 54% (13/24) ($p = 0.043$) in patients treated later.

Reduction in infarct size, as assessed by enzyme release (area under curve of enzyme plasma concentration against time), is apparently greater in patients treated earlier. Data from the ISAM trial are shown in Figure 5.[13] In that study randomization to streptokinase vs placebo was stratified according to DOT < or > 3 hours. Patients seen after 6 hours were not eligible. Simoons *et al.*[14] found a similar, although not significant, trend.

As far as left ventricular function is concerned, a trend has been observed for better recovery with patients treated earlier. Mathey *et al.* have compared pre-treatment values with values obtained 2–3 weeks after treatment:[15] the gain in regional hypokinasia was greater in patients treated earlier (DOT < 2 hours) than in patients treated later (DOT > 2 hours), (Fig. 6); the gain in global left ventricular ejection fraction was also greater (Fig. 7). In ISAM, coronary angiography was performed in a large sub-group of patients at 3–4 weeks after treatment. The global left ventricular ejection fraction was significantly greater in streptokinase treated patients as compared with the placebo group ($p < 0.01$) for those treated

Table 1 *Reperfusion rate and DOT in eight series of intravenous administration of streptokinase*

	%Reperfusion	*Delay (h)*	*Number of patients*
Blunda[6]	66.7	3.8	12
TIMI-1a[7]	43.9	3.0	41
TIMI-1b	24.3	5.7	78
Spann[12]	48.8	3.4	43
Hillis[8]	41.2	4.5	34
Neuhaus[9]	66.7	3.6	9
Schroeder a [11]	77.8	2.3	9
Schroeder b	33.3	4.6	12
Rogers[10]	30.8	6.5	26
Alderman[5]	61.5	3.4	13

before the third hour. The difference was not significant for those with DOT > 3 hours (Fig. 8).

More direct evidence from randomized clinical trials with i.v. thrombolysis

Data from randomized clinical trials with mortality as the main criterion of efficacy are the basis for more direct evidence.[13, 16–22] In all studies, sub-group analyses were performed relating to DOT. In all but two (AIMS and the European Working Group Trial) a lower DOT was associated with greater values for mortality risk reduction as well as lower p-values for comparisons between treated and control groups (Table 2). It should be pointed out that few trials have recruited patients after 6–12 hours. So data for longer DOTs are scarce.

These data were pooled and submitted to a non-linear weighed regression analysis (Fig. 9). A clear curvilinear relationship between risk reduction and DOT was apparent, even when the later findings from ISIS-2 are incorporated:

$$\ln(1-\text{risk}) = -0.28 \ln(\text{DOT}) - 0.08 \quad (p<0.02) \qquad (2)$$

Clearly this plausible – though as yet unproven – relationship deserves attention. No clinical trial has been designed specifically to address it. At the present time, the evidence for an inverse relationship between benefit and DOT after thrombolysis is based on only indirect evidence.

Table 2 *Risk ratio and DOT in eight RCT of thrombolytic agents against placebo where such are available. The lower figure in each cell is for the number of patients.*

<table>
<tr><th>DOT (hours)</th><th>0–1</th><th>1–2</th><th>2–3</th><th>3–4</th><th>4–5</th><th>5–6</th><th>6–7</th><th>7–8</th><th>8–9</th><th>9–12</th><th>12–24</th></tr>
<tr><td>AIMS</td><td colspan="4">0.58
660</td><td colspan="2">0.45
344</td><td colspan="5"></td></tr>
<tr><td>ISAM</td><td colspan="3">0.81
940</td><td colspan="3">0.89
770</td><td colspan="5"></td></tr>
<tr><td>WWIV-SK</td><td colspan="3">0.45
194</td><td colspan="3">0.99
174</td><td colspan="5"></td></tr>
<tr><td>GISSI-1</td><td>0.53
1277</td><td colspan="2">0.86
4817</td><td colspan="3">0.83
3649</td><td colspan="3">0.89
1352</td><td>1.16
594</td><td></td></tr>
<tr><td>ISIS-2</td><td>0.60
714</td><td>0.65
1908</td><td>0.70
2486</td><td>0.68
2369</td><td colspan="6">0.86
7269</td><td>0.80
2451</td></tr>
<tr><td>ECS-SK</td><td colspan="6">0.60
105</td><td colspan="2">0.57
97</td><td colspan="3">0.35
78</td></tr>
<tr><td>ASSET</td><td colspan="3">0.75
1971</td><td colspan="2">0.76
2992</td><td colspan="6"></td></tr>
<tr><td>ECSG-rtPA</td><td colspan="3">0.18
386</td><td colspan="3">0.90
335</td><td colspan="5"></td></tr>
</table>

Earlier treatment: pre-hospital treatment

DOTs are quite variable between institutions (Fig. 10). A median DOT of 4 hours was observed in the EMIP Pilot Study when data collected prospectively from eight cities in Europe were pooled (Fig. 11).[24] In that survey, patients first seen outside hospital could have received treatment two hours earlier (difference of median DOTs). The components of DOT were analysed in a trial, MEXAP, in which a comparison was made of pre-hospital administration of an antiarrhythmic agent and placebo in patients developing a MI.[29] Although the duration of components after delay may vary, the findings have one important feature in common (Fig. 12). The longest component is calling the ambulance. Making patients more aware of the possible implications of chest pain would have a major impact on the whole of the DOT. Nevertheless the first mandatory step to reduce dramatically the DOT is to shift administration of the thrombolytic agent from hospital ward to the spot where the patient is first seen by a medical team.

The potential benefit of pre-hospital administration of thrombolytic compared with in-hospital administration will depend on five factors (Figs 13 and 14):

1. The slope and the curvilinearity of the risk reduction – DOT function;
2. The delay between onset of symptoms and pre-hospital intervention;
3. The time gained over in-hospital intervention;
4. The percentage of patients who would have been eligible for in-hospital thrombolysis were the pre-hospital intervention not a current practice;
5. The cut-off DOT for in-hospital thrombolysis. [In many hospitals patients arrive late, after the cut-off DOT, and are not given thrombolytic agents.]

It should be stressed that a consequence of factor (2) is that small but easily achieved reductions in DOT should result in large gains in risk reduction.

Pre-hospital thrombolysis: unknown benefit/risk ratio

Even assuming that the curve of Figure 9 is valid, pre-hospital administration of a thrombolytic agent could confer more harm than benefit compared with in-hospital intervention.
The theoretical advantages of pre-hospital thrombolysis are:

1. A greater mortality risk reduction, assuming the hypothetical curve of Figure 9 is true;
2. An increased target population in those areas where doctors still fear that thrombolysis beyond some arbitrary DOT is more harmful than beneficial.

Potential adverse effects of such a strategy could, however, outweigh these theoretical advantages:

1. By increasing the number of patients with an incorrect diagnosis of MI; they will be subjected to the potential hazards of thrombolysis without the potential for benefit; in addition the total cost of care will increase with no commensurate gains;
2. By increasing the severity of adverse effects of thrombolysis.

The diagnosis of MI very early after the onset of symptoms is generally regarded as difficult, though no good evidence for this belief seems to exist. Moreover, the facilities available at home or in the ambulance for monitoring patients are inferior to those available in the coronary care unit; this has a bearing on diagnosis as well as on care. Allergic reactions, hypotension, ventricular arrhythmias, and bleeding are the most common adverse effects of thrombolytic agents; when they occur in a coronary care unit with adequately trained numbers of staff and sufficient monitoring and care facilities, experience has shown that total recovery is the rule except for patients with intracranial bleeding. Hence, fatalities due to adverse reaction may well increase with pre-hospital thrombolysis due to difficulties in the management of adverse reactions.

In summary, despite the hypothesis of a greater benefit with pre-hospital thrombolysis, its true benefit/risk ratio is still unknown.

The European Myocardial Infarction Project

Two series of pre-hospital thrombolysis have been reported [27, 28] as well as a small scale feasibility randomized trial.[9,10] In order to investigate the value of pre-hospital thrombolysis, a randomized trial has been set up under the aegis of the European Community. Anistreplase (APSAC) has been selected because it is the most easy thrombolytic agent to administer.

The effect of pre-hospital treatment on 30 days and long term survival is the primary objective of the study, with safety of the treatment and organizational feasibility at the Community level as secondary objectives. The study is a multicentre, randomized, double-blind placebo controlled trial. Eligible patients should have typical chest pain, ECG patterns suggestive of an evolving myocardial infarction or strong evidence of acute coronary heart disease, with no contra-indications to the treatment. More than 10,000 patients will be randomized at home or in the ambulance to either fibrinolytic treatment (i.v. anistreplase), or placebo. On admission to hospital, the patient will receive the alternative treatment (i.e. anistreplase for those who received placebo at home or in the ambulance and placebo for those who received anistreplase). Events and complications occurring during the pre-hospital and hospital phases will be recorded. Post-discharge mortality will be recorded through government agencies. In each city, a study coordinator will be responsible for the coordination of all the operations at the city level (recruitment and follow-up of patients, collection of study data). Throughout the study, the results will be monitored, under the direction of the policy board, with pre-determined rules. It is anticipated that recruitment will last 12 to 18 months. Survival status of all patients will be assessed after the inclusion of the last patient.

Conclusion

If it can ascertained that pre-hospital thrombolysis is more beneficial and cost-effective than hospital intervention, the care strategy for patients with AMI may change dramatically. This could be a real challenge in terms of public health.

References

1. Reimer KA, Lowe J E, Rasmussen M M, Jennings R B, The wavefront phenomenon of ischemic cell death. 1. Myocardial infarct size vs duration of coronary occlusion in dogs. *Circulation 56*, 1977, 786–794.
2. Chandler A B, Chapman I, Erhardt L R, Roberts W C, Schwartz C J, Sinapius D, Spain D M, Sherry S, Ness P, Simon T L, Coronary thrombosis in myocardial infarction. Report of a workshop of the role of coronary thrombosis in the pathogenesis of acute myocardial infarction. *Amer. J. Cardiol. 34*, 1974, 823–832.
3. Stehbens W.E, Relationship of coronary-artery thrombosis to myocardial infarction. *Lancet 2* 1985, 639–642.
4. Kennedy J W, Gensini G G, Timmis G C, Maynard C, Acute myocardial infarction treated with intracoronary streptokinase: a report of the society for cardiac angiography. *Amer. J. Cardiol 55*, 1985, 871–877.

5. Alderman E L, Jutzy K R, Berte L E, Miller R G, Friedman J P, Creger W P, Eliastam M, Randomized comparison of intravenous versus intracoronary streptokinase for myocardial infarction. *Amer. J. Cardiol 54*, 1984, 14–19.
6. Blunda M, Meister S G, Shechter J A, Pickering N J, Wolf N M, Intravenous versus intracoronary streptokinase for acute transmural myocardial infarction, *Catheter. Cardiovasc. Diagnosis 10*, 1984, 319–327.
7. Chesebro J H, Knatterud G, Roberts R, Borer J, Cohen L S, Dalen J, Dodge H T, Francis C K, Hillis D, Ludbrook P, Markis J E, Mueller H, Passamani E R, Powers E R, Rao A K, Robertson T, Ross A, Ryan T J, Sobel B E, Willerson J, Williams D O, Zaret B L, Braunwald E, Thrombolysis in Myocardial Infarction (TIMI) Trial, Phase I: a comparison between intravenous tissue plasminogen activator and intravenous streptokinase. *Circulation 76*, 1987, 142–154.
8. Hillis L D, Borer J, Braunwald E, Chesebro J H, Cohen L S, Dalen J, Dodge H T, Francis C K, Knatterud G, Ludbrook P, Markis J E, Mueller H, Desvig Ne-Nickens P, Passamani E R, Powers E R, Rao A K, Roberts R, Roberts W C, Ross A, Ryan T J, Sobel B E, High dose intravenous streptokinase for acute myocardial infarction: preliminary results of a multicenter trial. *J.A.C.C. 6*, 1985, 957–962.
9. Neuhaus K L, Kostering H, Tebbe U, Sauer G, Kreuzer H, Intravenose kurzzeit-streptokinase-therapie beim frischen myokardinfarkt. *Z. Kardiol 70*, 1981, 791–796.
10. Rogers W J, Mantle J A, Hood W P, Baxley W A, Whitlow P L, Reeves R C, Soto B, Prospective randomized trial of intravenous and intracoronary streptokinase in acute myocardial infarction. *Circulation 68*, 1983, 1051–1061.
11. Schroeder R, Biamino G, Leitner E R, Linderer T, Bruggemann T, Heitz J, Vohringer H F, Wegscheider K, Intravenous short-term infusion of streptokinase in acute myocardial infarction. *Circulation 67*, 1983, 536–548.
12. Spann J F, Sherry S, Carabello B A, Denenberg B S, Mann R H, McCann W D, Gault J H, Gentzler R D, Belber A D, Maurer A H, Cooper E M, Coronary thrombosis in intravenous streptokinase in acute myocardial infarction: acute and follow-up studies. *Amer. J. Cardiol. 53*, 1984, 655–661.
13. The I.S.A.M. Study Group. A prospective trial of intravenous streptokinase in acute myocardial infarction (I.S.A.M.). Mortality, Morbidity, and Infarct Size at 21 Days. *N.Engl. J.Med., 314*, 1986, 1465–1471.
14. Simoons M L, Serruys P W, Van Den Brand M, Res J, Verheugt F W A, Kraus X H, Remme W J, Bar F, de Zwann C, Van Der Laarse A, Vermeer F, Lubsen J, Early thrombolysis in acute myocardial infarction: Limitation of infarct size and improved survival. *J.A.C.C. 7*, 1986, 717–728.
15. Mathey D G, Sheenan F H, Schofer J, Dodge H T, Time from onset of symptoms to thrombolytic therapy: A major determinant of myocardial salvage in patients with acute transmural infarction. *J.A.C.C. 6*, 1985, 518–525.
16. AIMS Trial Study Group. Effect of intravenous APSAC on mortality after acute myocardial infarction: Preliminary report of a placebo-controlled clinical trial. *Lancet 1*, 1988, 545–549.
17. European Working Party. Strepokinase in Recent Myocardial Infarction: A controlled Multicentre Trial. *Br. Med. J. 3*, 1971, 325–331.
18. European Cooperative Study Group for streptokinase treatment in acute myocardial infarction. Streptokinase in acute myocardial infarction. *N. Engl. J. Med. 301*, 1979, 797–802.
19. Gruppo Italiano per lo studio della Streptochinasi nell'Infarto Miocardico (GISSI). Long-term effects of intravenous thrombolysis in acute myocardial infarction: final report of the GISSI study. *Lancet 3*, 1987, 871–874.

20. ISIS-2 (Second International Study of Infarct Survival) Collaborative Group. Randomised trial of intravenous streptokinase oral aspirin, both, or neither among 17,187 cases of suspected acute myocardial infarction: ISIS-2 *Lancet 2*, 1988, 349–360.
21. Van de Werf F, Arnold A E R, For the European Cooperative Study Group for recombinant tissue type plasminogen activator. Intravenous tissue plasminogen activator and size of infarct, left ventricular function, and survival in acute myocardial infarction. *Br. Med. J. 297*, 1988, 1374–1378.
22. Wilcox R G, Olsson C G, Skene A M, Von Der Lippe G, Jensen G, Hamptom J R. for the ASSET Study Group. Trial of tissue plasminogen activator for mortality reduction in acute myocardial infarction. Anglo-Scandinavian Study of Early Thrombolysis (ASSET). *Lancet 3*, 1988, 525–530.
23. Weinstein J, Somerville N J, Treatment of myocardial infarction with intracoronary streptokinase: Efficacy and safety data from 209 United States cases in the Hoechst-Roussel registry. *Amer Heart J. 104*, 1982, 894–898.
24. Report of the European Myocardial Infarction Project (E.M.I.P.) Sub-committee. Potential time saving with pre-hospital intervention in acute myocardial infarction. *Eur. Heart J. 9*, 1988, 118–124.
25. Herve Ch, Gaillard M, Castaigne A, Jan F, Huguenard P, Thrombolysis at home. *Lancet 3*, 1987, 1278.
26. Herve Ch, Gaillard M, Castaigne A, Jan F, Huguenard P. (1987), Thrombolysis at home. *Lancet 3*, 1987, 1459.
27. Koren G, Weiss A T, Hasin Y, Appelbaum D, Welber S, Rozenman Y, Lotan C, Mozzeri M, Sapoznikov D, Luria M H, Gotsman M S, Prevention of myocardial damage in acute myocardial ischemia by early treatment with intravenous streptokinase. *N. Engl. J. Med. 313*, 1985, 1384–1389.
28. Villemant D, Barriot P, Riou B, Bodenan P, Brunet F, Noto R, Monsallier J F, Achievement of thrombolysis at home in case of Acute Myocardial Infarction. *Lancet 1*, 1987, 1459.
29. Lievre M, Peyrieux J C, Leizorovicz A, Andre-Fouet X, Boissel J P, and the MEXAP Research Group. Antiarrhythmic effects and tolerability of Mexiletine in patients with suspected acute myocardial infarction. *Drug Investigation*, 1990, accepted for publication.

Chapter 9

THROMBOSIS AND THROMBOLYSIS IN UNSTABLE ANGINA: PERSPECTIVES

M. L. Brochier

University Hospital, Tours, France

Introduction

During the period from January 1981 to January 1988, a total of 7382 patients were admitted to our Coronary Care Unit. Of these, 2005 were admitted for acute myocardial infarction (AMI) and 931 patients were considered to have unstable angina pectoris (UA) including severe new onset or progressive angina, and chest pain at rest associated with ECG changes. In-hospital mortality rate for all patients with AMI was 13.4% and for all patients with UA was 3.4% (p <0.001) (Fig. 1)

Acute Myocardial infarction		Unstable angina
n = 2005		no. = 931
Death 13.4%	$p < .001$	Death 3.4%

Figure 1 *Morbidity and mortality from coronary artery diseases in Tours 1981–1988 (number of admitted patients = 7382)*

Since 40 to 50% of AMI are preceded by a period of UA it is obvious that UA is a phase in the evolution of coronary artery disease that provides an opportunity for effective therapy that may improve survival rate. Moreover, patients with AMI develop irreversible myocardial damage whereas patients with UA have coronary artery lesions without myocardial necrosis. Therefore UA is considered to be mainly arterial disease whereas MI is considered to be both arterial and myocardial disease.

Nevertheless, the natural history of UA is not stereotyped. Plotnik compared the wide variety of UA syndromes to a ‘bag of worms’ that can include UA *de novo*, worsening effort angina, mixed effort and rest angina, exclusive rest angina, early post-infarction angina, intermediate syndrome, variant vasospastic angina and even non-Q wave MI.

Among the patients with all these syndromes there is a subgroup who have chest pain at rest associated with ST-T ECG changes and a poor short and long-term prognosis. They should be distinguished from patients with new onset or progressive angina who have a prognosis that is only slightly worse than that of patients with chronic stable angina (Figs 2 and 3). Patients with such severe UA are usually admitted to an intensive coronary care unit because they fail to improve with usual conventional medical treatment and because they are considered to be refractory. In such patients, thrombosis is believed to play a major role leading to the unstable

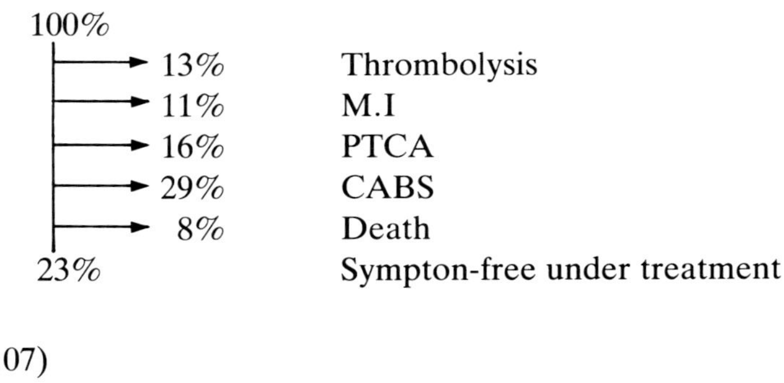

Figure 2 *In-hospital clinical course of unstable angina patients (Tours) (number of patients = 190)*

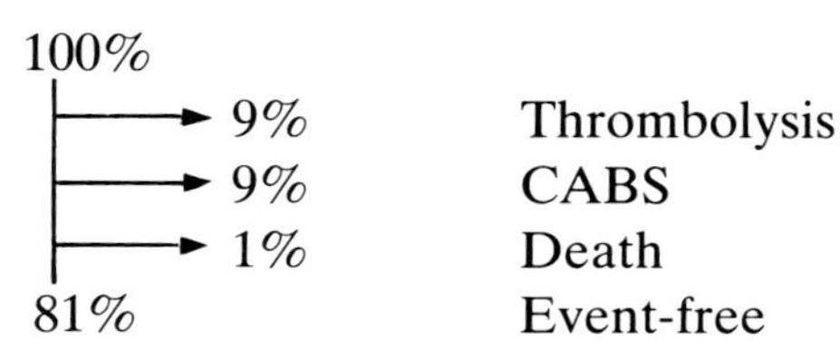

Figure 3 *Natural history and prognosis of unstable angina[19] (1980–1982), 28 day follow-up*

condition and usually to AMI and/or sudden death. Indeed, the role of intracoronary thrombus in this severe syndrome of UA has been demonstrated experimentally and pathologically, as well as by coronary angiography and angioscopy. Fuster[1] in the USA, and Davies[2] and Falk[3] in Europe have stressed the role of thrombosis in the evolution of coronary artery disease (CAD) (Fig. 4).

Experimental data

In experimental pig models,[4] the degree of vasospasm of a normal carotid artery after endothelial injury is proportional to the degree of platelet deposition at the site of injury. In concentrically narrowed canine coronary arteries, cyclic reductions in coronary flow have been demonstrated distal to the stenosis and appear to be related to platelet aggregation alternating with dislodgment of thrombus and embolization.[5]

Pathologic data

Microscopic examination of the coronary stenosis responsible for UA usually reveals a ruptured plaque surface (irregular stenosis) frequently associated with hemorrhage into the plaque and/or mural thrombosis leading to a rapid plaque progression. The thrombus adheres to the rupture

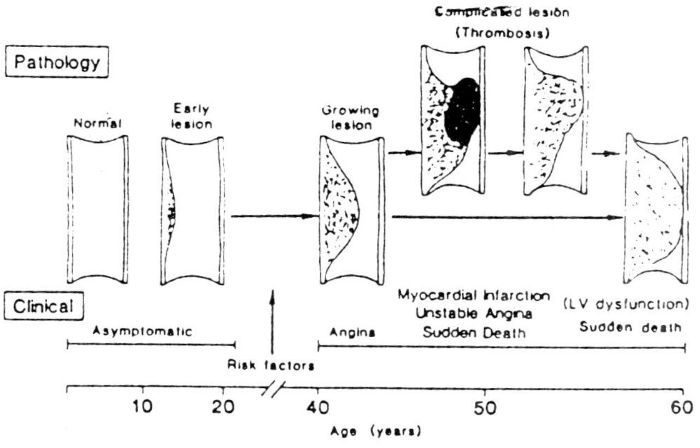

Figure 4 *Clinical and pathological evolution in coronary atherosclerotic disease (from Fuster, 1985)*

site where thrombogenic subendothelial tissue has been exposed and it may project into the lumen. Most interesting is the fact that the thrombus is usually layered, indicating intermittent growth by repeated mural deposits, and thrombus or microemboli are often found distally to the stenotic lesion (Fig. 5).[3] The thrombus formation at the rupture site is a dynamic process. The most recent part of the thrombus consists of aggregated platelets whereas older parts of the thrombus are infiltrated and stabilized by fibrin. In 1984, Davies[2] concluded that virtually all patients who die suddenly of ischaemic heart disease have actively progressing arterial lesions that are predominantly thrombotic.

Angiographic and angioscopic data

The pathologic findings in patients dying from UA correlate well with coronary angiography and angioscopy data as demonstrated by Ambrose[6] and Sherman.[7] Ambrose defines UA as only Class III or IV angina or prolonged rest pain that has recently increased by at least two

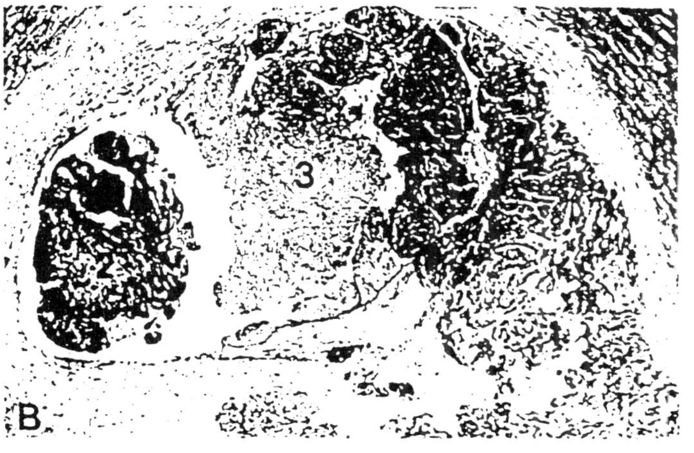

Figure 5 *Occlusive intracoronary thrombus formed in three stages in a case of unstable angina autopsy (from Falk, 1987)*

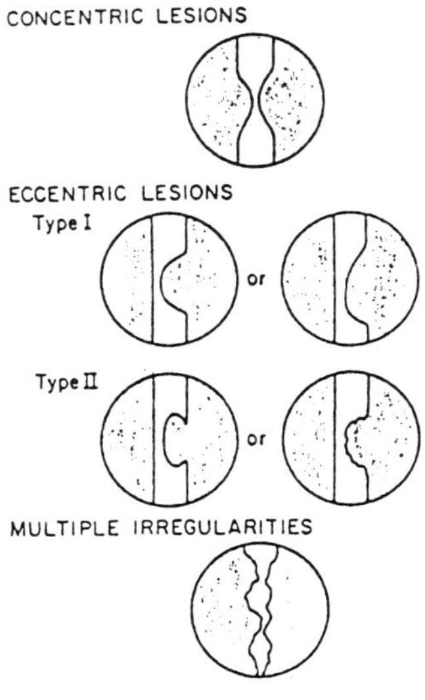

Figure 6 *Morphology of coronary lesions in acute coronary syndromes (from Ambrose, 1986)*

steps in the Canadian Heart Association Classification.[8] By qualitative analysis of coronary lesions in UA he found a characteristic eccentric lesion (type II eccentric and irregular lesion) in two-thirds of patients (Fig. 6). This kind of coronary lesion is common in an acute presentation of UA, recent non-Q wave infarction, acute MI with ST segment elevation or recent Q wave MI whereas it is rarely found in patients with stable angina. It is likely that the type II eccentric lesion represents a disrupted plaque or a partially occlusive thrombus or both.

In 1985, Capone *et al.*[9] reported the frequency of intracoronary filling defects by angiography in patients with detected angina at rest. Intracoronary thrombi were found in none of 35 patients with stable angina whereas they were detected in 37% of 119 patients with UA. Moreover they were present in 52% of patients when coronary arteriography was performed within 24 hours after the last rest pain and in 28% when coronary arteriography was performed later on within two weeks. Thus intracoronary thrombi were common in patients with UA who had active symptoms, and preliminary data with angioscopic technique have shown that thrombi (and/or plaque rupture) are more frequent even than suggested by angiography. The filling defects in UA are located either within or distal to the culprit lesion. Within the lesion, the filling defect probably represents thrombus at the site of a disrupted atherosclerotic plaque whereas distal to a

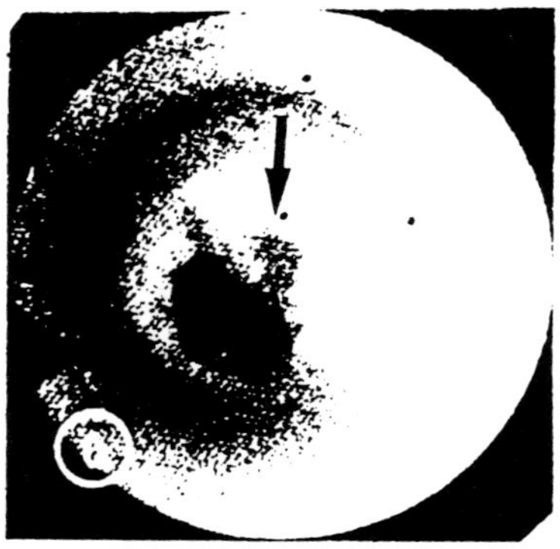

Figure 7 *Thrombus formation, a severe spasm in spastic coronary segment (from Uchida, 1987)*

Table 1 *Reduction of coronary events and death in unstable angina patients treated with aspirin (from Lewis, 1983). Veterans Administration Cooperative Study in 1266 patients with UA, AMI in 12 week follow-up.*

	No. of patients		*Reduction*	
Event	*Placebo (n=641)*	*Aspirin (n=625)*	*In aspirin group %*	*p Value*
Death or AMI	65(10.1)	31(5.0)	51	0.0002
Fatal or non-fatal MI	50(7.8)	22(3.5)	55	0.0003
Non-fatal MI	44(6.9)	21(3.4)	51	0.002

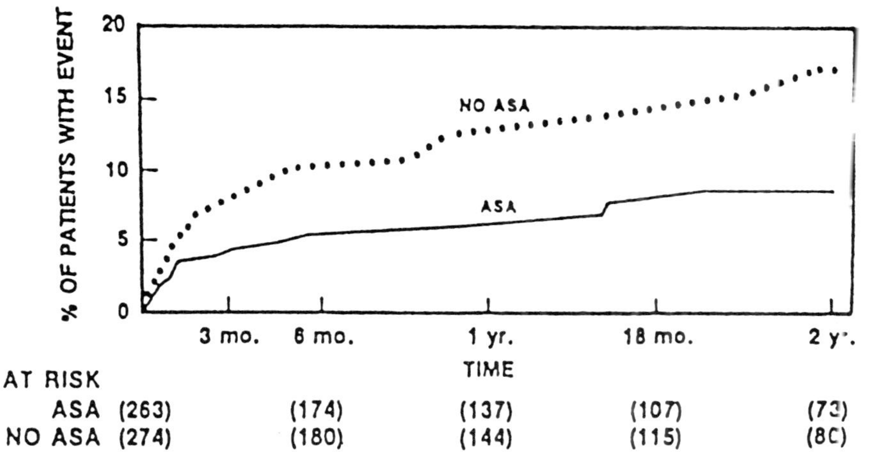

Figure 8 *Efficacy of ASA versus no ASA in reducing cardiac death or non-fatal myocardial infarction in patients with unstable angina (from Cairns, 1985)*

Table 2 *Time related intracoronary thrombi in unstable angina patients*

	No.	*Delay pain–angio* Days	*thrombus+* N	%
Vetrovec (1981)	129	30	8	6.2
Vetrovec (1982)	12	5	10	85
Zack (1984)	83	12–90	10	12
Capone (1985)	44	<1	23	52
	75	<14	21	28
Gotho (1985)	18	<1	8	44
	39	2	22	56
Brochier (1988)	20	<2	7	35
Gotho (1988)	37	0	21	57

lesion it probably represents a thrombus formation due to altered flow patterns with reduced or turbulent blood flow.

Angioscopy in patients with UA was performed by Sherman in 1986[7] (Fig. 7) during coronary artery bypass surgery. He identified thrombi in the offending vessel in all seven patients of the series with angina at rest refractory to medical treatment whereas none of the patients with stable coronary disease had either a complex plaque or thrombus. The thrombi varied from partially to completely occlusive and were often detected on the distal (downstream) side of an arterial obstruction at angiography. He concluded that ragged, ulcerated, haemorrhagic endothelium and acute thrombi characterize the coronary artery independently identified as causing the acute ischaemic syndrome and he suggested 'the need for systematic investigation of the risks and benefits of anticoagulant, antiplatelet, and thrombolytic therapy in patients with unstable coronary syndromes'.

Therapeutic implications

Antithrombotic Therapy in UA

Antiplatelet drugs, which can prevent platelet aggregation, do not prevent the attachment of the single layer of platelets, as pointed out by Lam.[4] Clinical trials in UA[10, 11] demonstrated that aspirin therapy was able to reduce both myocardial infarction and death but did not reduce the frequency of angina attacks. This is consistent with the experimental evidence that eliminate arterial vasospasm (Table 1 and Fig 8).

Recently Theroux *et al.*[12] compared heparin alone (5,000 U as a bolus followed by an infusion of 1,000 U per hour) with aspirin alone (650 mg orally followed by 325 mg twice daily) and with both treatments in a similar dosage in 479 randomized patients with UA within 8 hours after last chest pain. Heparin was associated with a decrease in the occurrence of refractory angina. The incidence of MI was significantly reduced in the three groups and no death occurred within 1 week. But there was a trend favouring heparin over aspirin and the combination of the two drugs had no greater protective effect than heparin alone.

Thrombolysis in UA

The literature shows that the frequency of intracoronary thrombosis in UA depends first on the type of syndrome; it is rarely present in severe effort angina but is frequent in prolonged chest pain at rest with ST-segment changes. Secondly the frequency of thrombosis is time-related when assessed by coronary angiography and varies from 6% after one month to 57% when coronary arteriography is performed during chest pain (Table 2). Nevertheless two facts remain to be defined more accurately: the frequency of thrombotic material at the site of eccentric irregular coronary lesions (type II B of Ambrose) and the efficacy of thrombolytic treatment in acute refractory UA.

In 1987, a pilot study was conducted in our institution to assess both the frequency of thrombosis and the risk benefit of thrombolytic treatment in patients admitted to the intensive coronary care unit of Tours with UA. Inclusion criteria were age below 75 years, recent onset of UA (less than 3 weeks), prolonged chest pain at rest (> 15 min < 30 min) and transient ST segment and/or wave change. Exclusion criteria were a recent MI, abnormal increase of CK level, contraindications to thrombolytic treatment, and the lack of feasibility of coronary angiogram before and after treatment.

After the initial coronary angiogram, patients with left main coronary artery stenosis or with normal coronary angiogram, were excluded from treatment. Thrombolytic therapy was started immediately after the initial coronary angiogram and the second coronary angiogram was performed within 36 hours after treatment. All coronary angiograms were evaluated first locally and then centrally by quantitative analysis using the CASS system.

All patients were given conventional treatment and full heparinization and had serial biological controls for enzymes and coagulation parameters. From the 20 patients included in the study, four patients were excluded after the initial coronary angiogram because two had left main coronary artery stenosis and two had contra-indications to thrombolysis. 16 patients were given thrombolytic therapy, and 14 had the two coronary angiograms before and after treatment (two were excluded from the second coronary angiogram because of bleeding complications).

The summarized results were as follows:

– Intracoronary thrombi were present in seven out of 20 patients (35%): one was occlusive and 6 non occlusive. The frequency was higher (67%) for the nine patients who had a coronary angiogram within 12 hours of chest pain than for the 11 patients who had a coronary angiogram after the 12th hour (9%).
– The efficacy of thrombolytic therapy in the seven cases of intracoronary thrombi was slight since only one thrombus totally disappeared, four thrombi (one occlusive, three non occlusive) were unchanged and two non occlusive thrombi were reduced by thrombolytic therapy.
– Arterial stenosis was present in 17 out of 20 cases, associated with intracoronary thrombi in six cases and without any thrombus in 11 cases. Ten of 17 artery stenoses were **eccentric** and **irregular**, type II B of Ambrose (59% of cases). After the second coronary angiogram (n = 14), none of the stenoses had changed either on visual assessment, or with quantitative assessment.
– Moreover, plaque area (mm^2) and stenosis diameter (%) which are the most sensitive variables studied by the CASS system did not change beyond the confidence limits.

The in-hospital course included:

– Emergency percutaneous transluminal coronary angioplasty (PTCA) n = 3;

Figure 9 *PTCA in unstable angina. Cumulative incidence of coronary events (from de Feyter et al., JACC 12*, 1988, 324–333)

n = 200

	Function Class I	Death	Primary success	MI	CABG
Early	0	0.5%	89.5%	8%	9%
6 Mths			Restenosis 51/158		
	89%	1.5%	32%	95%	13%
2 Yrs			re-PTCA 23/196		
	86%	3%	12%	12%	15%

– Fatal myocardial infarction n = 1;
– Recurrent ischaemia (n = 4) treated with two PTCA and two coronary artery by-pass grafts (CABG);
– Stabilization (n = 8) (4 of them had only medical treatment, the three others needed elective PTCA (n = 2) and elective CABG (n = 2)

Bleeding complications occurred in four out of 16 thrombolysed patients, two moderate and two severe (one cerebrovascular haemorrhage, one acute renal failure).

During mean follow-up of 12 months (range 6–8 months) all eight medical and CABG patients were asymptomatic with negative stress test; all seven PTCA patients were asymptomatic, nevertheless one of them had positive stress test, angiographic restenosis and secondary CABG.

Comments

These results are consistent with existing data in the literature.

1. Intracoronary thrombosis is frequent in UA patients who are seen soon after rest pain (67% in patients before the 12th hour).

2. Success rate of thrombolysis on intracoronary thrombi is 43% in this short series. It is low in the literature by comparison with reperfusion rate in AMI and with the success rate of PTCA in UA (85–90%). This is not surprising since thrombosis might have been present for a longer time in UA than in AMI.

3. Thrombolyis does not seem to improve the stenosis diameter of the ischaemia related artery since no changes were observed by quantitative assessment of the culprit lesions in our series or in the study of Topol after rt-PA.[13]

4. After thrombolytic therapy, eight out of 16 patients (50%) became asymptomatic but thrombolysis did not prevent ischaemic recurrences in 56% of cases and did not reduce significantly the need for further revascularization, as in the study of Zwaan.[14] In these patients

treated by previous full heparinization, bleeding complications were frequent (25%) as in the series of gold.[15]

5. Thrombolysis can be compared with early PTCA and/or CABG in this variety of severe UA patients. Although the initial success rate of PTCA is much higher (85–90%), the risks of the procedure in the acute setting are rather high[16] with 0.5% mortality, 8% with MI, 9% having emergency CABG (Fig. 9). The alternative of coronary bypass surgery is also associated with a rather high complication rate[17] and an operative mortality rate of 5.3% in the special subset of patients with unstable post-infarction angina.[18]

6. Finally thrombolysis should be limited to selected cases of patients with UA at rest that is refractory to medical treatment. More controlled prospectives studies with fibrin-specific agents are required to assess both efficacy and risk–benefit ratio of thrombolysis in UA. With rt-PA the need for PTCA was eliminated in a few patients in the study of Topol[13] and the safety of PTCA was improved.

In France, two multicenter randomized placebo-controlled studies are ongoing using either rt-PA or APSAC in selected UA patients.

Conclusion

It is likely that thrombolytic therapy will have a place in the future for patients with prolonged and refractory unstable angina at rest. The time efficacy of thrombolysis in these acute coronary syndromes has not been yet established, however, and needs further evaluation.

References

1. Fuster V, Steele P M, Chesebro J H, Role of platelets and thrombosis in coronary atherosclerotic disease and sudden death. *J. Am. Coll. Cardiol. 5*, 1985, 175 B.
2. Davies M J, Thomas A, Thrombosis and acute coronary artery lesions in sudden cardiac ischemic death. *N. Engl. J. Med. 310*, 1984, 1137–1140.
3. Falk E, Plaque rupture with severe pre-existing stenosis precipitating coronary thrombosis. Characteristics of coronary atherosclerotic plaques underlying fatal occlusive thrombi. *Br. Heart J. 50*, 1983 127–134.
4. Lam J Y T, Chesebro J H, Steele P M, Badimon L, Fuster V, Is vasospasm related to platelet deposition? Relationship in a porcine preparation of arterial injury *in vivo*. *Circulation 75*, 1987, 243–248.
5. Folts J D, Gallagher K, Rowe G G, Blood flow reductions in stenosed canine coronary arteries: vasospasm or platelet aggregation? *Circulation 65*, 1982, 248–255.
6. Ambrose J A, Winters S L, Stern A, Teichholz L E, Gorlin R, Fuster V, Angiographic morphology and the pathogenesis of unstable angina pectoris. *J. Amer. Coll. Cardiol. 5*, 1985, 609–616.
7. Sherman C T, Litvack F, Grundfest W, Lee M, Hickey A, Chaux A, Kass R, Blanche C, Matloff J, Morgenstern L, Ganz W, Swan H J C, Forrester J, Coronary angioscopy in patients with unstable angina pectoris. *New Engl. J. Med. 315*, 1986, 915–919.
8. Ambrose J A, Winters S L, Arora R R, Eng A, Riccio A, Gorlin R, Fuster V, Angiographic evolution of coronary artery morphology in unstable angina. *J. Amer. Coll. Cardiol. 7*, 1986, 472–478.
9. Capone G, Wolf N M, Meyer B, Meister S G, Frequency of intracoronary filling defects by angiography in angina pectoris at rest. *Am. J. Cardiol. 56*, 1985, 403–406.
10. Lewis H D, Davies J W, Archibald D G *et al.*, Protective effects of aspirin against acute myocardial infarction and death in man with unstable angina. *N. Engl. J. Med. 309*, 1983, 396–403.

11. Cairns J A, Gent M, Singer J *et al.* Aspirin, sulfinpyrazone or both in unstable angina: results of a Canadian multicenter trial. *N. Engl. J. Med. 313*, 1985, 1369–1375.
12. Theroux P, Quimet H, McCans J, Latour J G, Joly P, Levy G, Pelletier E, Juneau M, Stasiak J, de Guise P, Pelletier G B, Rinzler D, Waters D D, Aspirin, heparin or both to treat acute unstable angina. *N. Engl. J. Med. 319*, 1988, 1105–1111.
13. Topol E J, Nicklas J M, Kander N H, Walton J A, Ellis S G, Gorman L, Pitt B, Coronary revascularization after intravenous tissue plasminogen activator for unstable angina pectoris: results of a randomized double-blind, placebo-controlled trial. *Amer. J. Cardiol. 62*, 1988, 368–371.
14. de Zwaan C, Bar F W, Janssen J H A, de Swart H B, Vermeer F, Wellens H J J, Effects of thrombolytic therapy in unstable angina: clinical and angiographic results. *J. Amer. Coll. Cardiol. 12*, 1988, 301–309.
15. Gold H K, Johns J A, Leinbach R C, Yasuda T, Collen D, Thrombolytic therapy for unstable angina: rationale and results. *J. Amer. Coll. Cardiol. 10*, 1987, 91B-5B
16. de Feyter, Suryapranata H, Serruys P W, Beatt K, van Domburg R, van der Brand M, Tijssen J J, Azar, A J, Hugenholtz P G, Coronary angioplasty for unstable angina: immediate and late results in 200 consecutive patients with identification of risk factors for unfavorable early and late outcome. *J. Amer. Coll. Cardiol. 12*, 1988, 324–333.
17. Luchi R J, Scott S M, Dupree R H, Comparison of medical and surgical treatment for unstable angina pectoris. Results of a Veterans' Administration Cooperative Study. *N. Engl. J. Med. 316*, 1987, 977–984.
18. Scott S M, Luchi R J, Deupree R H and the Veterans' Administration Unstable Angina Cooperative Study Group – Veterans' Administration Cooperative Study for treatment of patients with unstable angina. Results in patients with abnormal left ventricular function. *Circulation 78*, 1988, I.113–I.121
19. Mulcahy R, Al Awadhi A H, de Buitleor M, Tobin G, Johnson H, Contoy R, Natural history and prognosis of unstable angina. *Am. Heart J. 109*, 1985, 753–758.

Chapter 10

THE DEVELOPMENT OF A SECOND GENERATION TISSUE PLASMINOGEN ACTIVATOR

Edward F. Fritsch, Jay Stoudemire, Gregg Timony, Patricia Horgan and Glenn R. Larsen

Genetics Institute, Cambridge, MA, USA

Introduction

Tissue-type plasminogen activator (t-PA) is a glycoprotein in the plasminogen activator family that activates the zymogen plasminogen to the protease plasmin (see reference 1 for review). Plasmin is an important protease active in the degradation of fibrin clots. The conversion of plasminogen to plasmin by t-PA is catalyzed selectively on fibrin clots. Thus, t-PA has been regarded as a promising therapeutic with potentially reduced side effects. Recently, recombinant t-PA has been approved for treatment of acute myocardial infarction, based on its fibrinolytic activity and its ability to improve left ventricular function.

The current recommended doses for t-PA are 100 mg administered by constant intravenous infusion as 60 mg during the first hour, 20 mg over the second hour and 20 mg over the third hour. This dosing regimen is primarily a consequence of the pharmacokinetic profile of t-PA, which is characterized by a rapid and predominant initial alpha phase (t 1/2 = ~6 minutes in man), followed by a more prolonged beta phase representing only a small proportion of the protein.[2] Because of the rapid alpha phase, the protein must be continually supplied in order to maintain a therapeutic level in the circulation.

The primary objective of our work has been the identification of a variant molecule that could be delivered by a single bolus injection and be efficacious in lysing arterial clots. Our approach to achieving this objective was to define variants of t-PA that had significantly improved half-lives relative to wild type t-PA. In addition to permitting bolus delivery, it is possible that a longer lived molecule would also require a lower total dose, thus potentially reducing side effects, cost, or both. The biochemical and pharmacological (pharmacokinetics and efficacy) profiles of some of these variants have been carried out and will be discussed below.

Materials and methods

The wild type t-PA and variant t-PAs used in these studies were produced in Chinese hamster ovary cells as described previously.[3,4] All biochemical procedures have been previously described.[3,4] Details of the rabbit pharmacokinetic and clot lysis experiments are presented in the figure legends.

Results

Deletion of the finger and EGF (epidermal growth factors) domains of wild type t-PA

t-PA is a multi-domain molecule, consisting of five distinct domains (fibronectin finger-like domain, epidermal growth factor-like domain, two kringle domains, and the serine protease domain). In an attempt to define whether any of these domains were individually responsible for the rapid clearance of wild type t-PA, site directed mutagenesis was carried out. Initially the finger and epidermal growth factor domains were deleted (residues Cys_6-Asn_{87}), resulting in the variant termed FE. In addition, separate deletions of the finger (Cys_6-Ser_{50}) and the epidermal growth factor (Cys_{51}-Asn_{87}) were also prepared, resulting in the F and E variants, respectively. Pharmacokinetic studies in rats using 35-S metabolically labeled proteins produced in CHO cells[5] indicated that the plasma radioactivity time curve of the FE variant could be described as a monophasic curve with a calculated half-life of 27 minutes (compared with a half-life of 0.8 minutes for the alpha phase of wild type t-PA in the same experiment). Results with the individual domain deletions (F and E) suggested that the deletion of the finger domain was primarily responsible for this effect since the plasma decay curve of the F variant was again monophasic with a calculated half-life of 17 minutes while the decay curve for the E variant was biphasic, the half-life of the alpha phase being only 2.1 minutes. Biochemical analysis of these variants[3] however, revealed that the affinity for fibrin for each of these variants was significantly reduced compared to wild type t-PA. In addition, at low plasminogen activator concentrations, the variants were less effective than wild type t-PA in clot lysis *in vitro* in human plasma, although at high concentrations (>l μg/ml), the *in vitro* fibrinolytic potential was improved compared to that of wild type t-PA. Thus, the FE deletion resulted in a variant t-PA with significantly improved pharmacokinetic properties but some evidence of an enzymatic defect, perhaps due to the reduction in fibrin affinity. Additional variants were then constructed to modify further these properties.

N-linked carbohydrate variants of FE t-PA

Studies with wildtype t-PA produced in Chinese hamster ovary (CHO) cells in the presence or absence of tunicamycin indicated that the absence of all N-linked carbohydrate on t-PA resulted in a molecule with significantly higher fibrin affinity and *in vitro* fibrinolytic activity.[4] Based on these results, the variant FE3X was constructed by site directed mutagenesis of Asn to Gln at each of the three N-linked glycosylation sites (positions 117, 184, and 448). In addition, to evaluate the significance of the 'high mannose' carbohydrate on the N-linked glycosylation site at position 117 and the possibility that receptors in the liver for high mannose carbohydrate might be a mechanism for clearance of t-PA, the variant FE1X was constructed by mutagenesis of Asn to Gln at position 117 only. The biochemical and pharmacokinetic properties of these variants were then compared.[4]

Fibrin binding studies with FE, FE1X, FE3X and wild type t-PA indicated that FE1X demonstrated a similar degree of reduction in fibrin binding as observed for FE while FE3X regained some but not all of the fibrin affinity of wild type t-PA. For FE3X, fibrin binding was similar to wild type t-PA at fibrin concentrations above 1 mg/ml but still significantly reduced below 0.2 mg/ml. When the variants were compared in *in vitro* clot lysis experiments, however, both FE1X and FE3X demonstrated better lysis at low plasminogen activator concentrations than FE but still less lysis than wild type t-PA. At higher concentrations (>1 μg/ml), the fibrinolytic activity of each of the variants was improved.

Pharmacokinetic studies of these variants following bolus injection in rats[5] or following discontinuation of constant intravenous infusion in rabbits[6] indicated that FE3X had a shorter half-life than either FE or FE1X. The more rapid half life of FE3X may be due to the substantial reduction in size and charge by removal of all the N-linked carbohydrate, resulting in more effective removal through the kidney. Consistent with this hypothesis is the observation that a greater proportion of FE3X is found in the kidney in tissue distribution studies.

Figure 1 shows the pharmacokinetic profiles of FE1X and FE3X compared with Activase following bolus injection in rabbits. Each of these plasminogen activators was injected at a dose

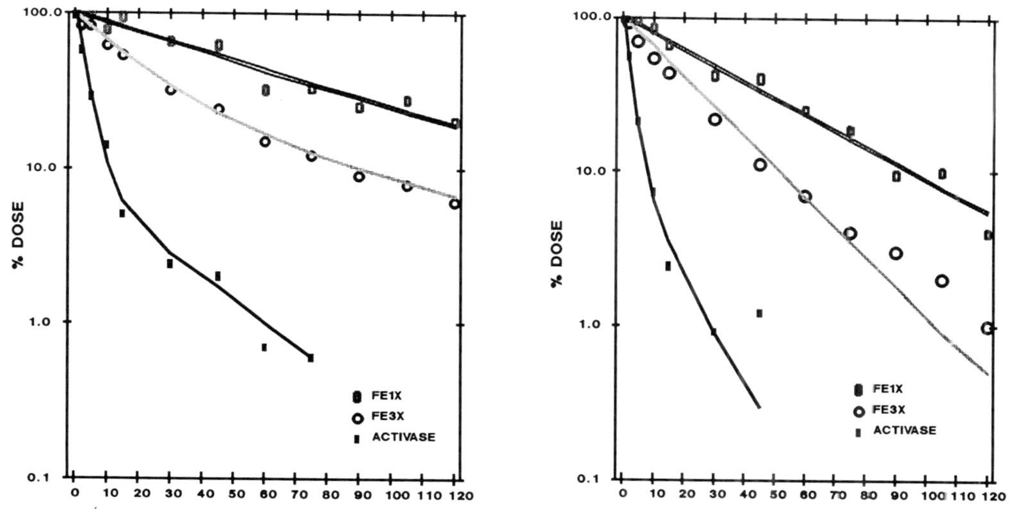

Figure 1 *Rabbits received a bolus injection through the marginal ear vein of unlabelled protein at a dose of 0.25 mg protein/kg body weight. Blood samples were taken at intervals following the injection and the t-PA antigen and activity levels were measured in plasma. Plasma antigen and activity time curves were constructed from these data and the curves were fitted to a multiexponential function of the form:* $C(t) = Ae^{-at} + Be^{-bt}$ *using a nonlinear curve-fitting program. Pharmacokinetic parameters (see Table 1) were estimated from these functions including area under the curve (AUC) and clearance from the plasma (Clp).*

of 0.25 mg/kg as a single bolus injection into the marginal ear vein and at the indicated times plasma samples were withdrawn through a femoral catheter and analyzed for t-PA antigen by ELISA and for activity by the S-2251 chromogenic substrate assay. Each data point is the mean of six individual rabbits. Activase was cleared more rapidly from the plasma than either FE1X or FE3X, while FE3X was cleared more rapidly than FE1X. A summary of these pharmacokinetic parameters is presented in Table 1. Compared with Activase, the relative decrease in clearance of the antigen and activity were approximately 18 to 20-fold for FE1X and 9-fold for FE3X.

Table 1 *Summary of pharmacokinetic parameters for t-PA and t-PA variants*

			Rabbit		
	Agent	*Dose (mg/kg)*	*Auc (ug min/ml)*	*Clearance (ml/min)*	*Clearance relative to activase*
Antigen					
	FE1X	0.25	651	1	18
	FE3X	0.25	309	2	9
	Activase	0.25	37	18	-
	Approximate concentration at T=0 : 5.6 μg/ml				
		Units/kg	μmin/ml		
Activity					
	FEIX	86,750	102,781	2	22
	FE3X	139,705	76,158	5	9
	Activase	176,250	10,583	44	-

The increases in area under the curve (AUC) were consistent with the decreased clearance. Interestingly the activity in the plasma decreased more rapidly than the antigen levels for each of the molecules. This difference may result from the inactivation of the protein after complexation with circulating inhibitors, assuming that such a complex was maintained in circulation and retained immunoreactivity.

In vivo clot lysis following bolus administration

To determine whether the reduced clearance rates and the reduced fibrin affinity of the variant proteins relative to wild type t-PA had an effect on *in vivo* clot lysis and to determine if the variants could be delivered by a single bolus dose and effectively lyse a clot, an *in vivo* thrombolysis model was set up based on the rabbit jugular vein model initially described by Collen *et al.*[7] The result of this study is presented in Figure 2 which presents the percent lysis as a function of dose. Control experiments to assess radioactivity washout and/or intrinsic fibrinolytic activity were carried out following injection of saline only. The background level was 11% ± 1% (SEM). At the lowest dose of Activase tested (0.063 mg/kg), the lysis was not significantly above background (10% ± 2%) while at the same dose level, FE3X resulted in approximately 25% lysis. At higher dose levels, FE3X consistently gave significantly greater lysis than Activase. Using 50% lysis to compare the potency of FE3X and Activase, FE3X is approximately 4-fold more potent. This result is consistent with previous studies in the dog using the copper coil-induced coronary artery thrombosis model.[8] In those studies FE3X was shown to have a higher thrombolytic efficacy than melanoma derived wild type t-PA following a single bolus administration.

Conclusions

Deletions of the finger and epidermal growth factor domains from wild type t-PA resulted in a molecule (FE) with improved pharmacokinetic properties but reduced fibrin binding. Elimination of all three N-linked carbohydrate addition sites from the FE deletion resulted in a molecule

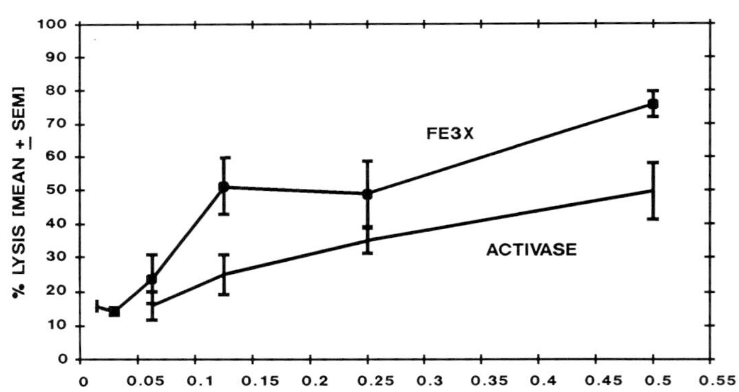

Figure 2 *The jugular vein of a rabbit was exposed and a small segment ligated off. Radioactive fibrinogen was added to whole rabbit blood, thrombin was added, and the mixture injected into the ligated segment to form a clot. Female rabbits of similar maturational age (12 weeks) were used for all these studies. The clot was allowed to mature for 30 minutes before the ligature was removed. Immediately after removal of the ligature, a single bolus dose of plasminogen activator was administered into the marginal ear vein. The dose was based on the weight of the rabbit and is expressed in mg protein/kg body weight. After 2 hours, the jugular vein segment containing the radioactive clot was excised and the amount of radioactivity was determined and expressed as percent lysis (percentage of input counts no longer present in the clot). Each thrombolytic agent (Activase, FE3X) was examined at multiple does levels in six rabbits at each dose.*

(FE3X) with a more rapid clearance compared with FE, but improvement in fibrin affinity. Elimination of the high mannose carbohydrate addition site resulted in a molecule (FE1X) with a half-life longer than that of FE3X but no improvement in fibrin binding over that of FE. *In vivo* clot lysis studies following single bolus injections of either wild type t-PA or the FE3X variant demonstrated superiority of the FE3X molecule over wild type t-PA. These studies thus support the development of variant forms of t-PA with increased half-lives as candidate second generation plasminogen activators to be tested clinically.

Reference

1. Loscalzo J, and Braunwald E, *N. Eng. J. Med. 319*; 1988, 925–931.
2. Verstraete M, Su C A P F, Tanswell P, Feuerer S A, and Collen D, *Thromb. Haemostasis 56*; 1986, 1–5.
3. Larsen G R, Henson K, Blue Y, *J. Biol. Chem. 263*; 1988, 1023–1029.
4. Hansen L, Blue Y, Barone K, Collen D, Larsen G R *J. Biol. Chem. 293*; 1988, 15713–15719.
5. Larsen G R, Metzger M, Henson K, Blue Y, Horgan P, *Blood 73*; 1989, 1842–1850.
6. Collen D, Stassen J M, Larsen G R, *Blood 71*; 1988, 216–219.
7. Collen D, Stassen J M, Verstraete M, *J. Clin. Invest. 71*; 1983, 368–376.
8. Cambier P, Van de Werf F, Larsen G R, Collen D, *J. Cardiovas. Pharm. 11*; 1988, 468–472.

Chapter 11

NEWER STRATEGIES IN ANTI-THROMBOTIC PATHWAYS – THROMBOXANE RECEPTOR ANTAGONISTS

Edward F. Smith III, Gregory A. Kopia, Eliot H. Ohlstein and Robert R. Ruffolo, Jr.

SmithKline Beecham Pharmaceuticals, plc, King of Prussia, PA, USA

Introduction

The role of thromboxane (TX) A_2 in pathophysiologic conditions has been an area of extensive investigation. TXA_2 is an enzymatic product of arachidonic acid metabolism that is formed from the prostaglandin endoperoxide intermediates, PGG_2 and PGH_2. The prerequisite enzymes responsible for TX formation are found abundantly in platelets and white cells, but blood vessels and other tissue also possess the capacity to synthesize TX. Biologically, TXA_2 is a potent contractile substance on vascular and pulmonary smooth muscle, a potent platelet aggregator, a membrane lytic agent, and may effect neutrophil adhesion. These properties of TXA_2 suggest an important role in various cardiovascular disorders including coronary artery thrombosis, coronary artery fibrinolysis, and myocardial reperfusion injury.

Initially, only cyclooxygenase and TX synthase inhibitors were available as tools to investigate the pharmacology and pathophysiology of TXA_2. However, both classes of agents have certain limitations. Recently, considerable progress has been made in the development of high affinity, selective TX receptor antagonists. The purpose of this review will be to summarize the evidence that TX receptor antagonists represent efficacious drugs for reducing the incidence of platelet-dependent coronary artery thrombosis, enhancing the efficacy of the fibrinolytic agents' tissue-type plasminogen activator (t-PA) and streptokinase, and reducing the extent of myocardial reperfusion injury.

Pharmacology of TXA_2

A number of different pharmacological agents are available with which to investigate the pathophysiology of TXA_2. These include cyclooxygenase inhibitors, TX synthase inhibitors and TX receptor antagonists. The cyclooxygenase inhibitors are generally known as the nonsteroidal, antiinflammatory drugs (NSAID), and include agents such as aspirin, indomethacin, and ibuprofen. The pharmacology of the cyclooxygenase inhibitors is generally well characterized, and both short and longer acting agents are available. However, a disadvantage of cyclooxygenase inhibitors is that they inhibit simultaneously the formation of both deleterious (i.e., TXA_2) and beneficial (i.e., PGI_2) products. Additionally, metabolism of arachidonic acid may be redirected towards the 5-lipoxygenase pathway. The nonselective inhibition of both TXA_2 and PGI_2, in addition to the 'shunting' of arachidonic acid metabolism to leukotriene products may not only complicate the interpretation of the mechanism of action of these drugs, but may also limit the efficacy of this class of agents.

The development of TX synthase inhibitors represented a more specific approach to inhibition of TX formation. The pharmacologic activities of most TX synthase inhibitors are well characterized, and most compounds are significantly more potent and selective than the prototypic inhibitor, imidazole. However, Smith *et al.*[1] reported that dazoxiben inhibited TX formation of thrombin-stimulated human platelets in a concentration-dependent fashion, but was completely without effect for preventing the contraction produced by addition of these stimulated platelets to isolated vascular segments. The TX receptor antagonist, sulotroban, and the NSAID, indomethacin, effectively blocked the vascular contraction elicited by thrombin-stimulated platelets.[2] These observations illustrate an important limitation of TX synthase inhibitors: that they do not prevent the formation or activity of the prostaglandin endoperoxides, PGG_2 and PGH_2, and may, in fact, redirect substrate towards other broncho- and vasoconstrictor agents (i.e., PGD_2 and $PGF_{2\alpha}$). A further concern with most TX synthase inhibitors studied to date is the short duration of action and the disappointing clinical efficacy.

Recently, a number of TX receptor antagonists have been developed and characterized. TX receptor antagonists are more useful than TX synthase inhibitors in assessing the effects of TX receptor activation, and for pharmacologic characterization of the TX receptor on platelets, vascular and other preparations.[4] Moreover, TX receptor antagonists do not alter arachidonic acid metabolism, and therefore the specific effects of TXA_2, *vis-à-vis* altered formation of other prostanoids, can be determined. Among the more commonly used agents with high affinity and specificity for the TX receptor are sulotroban (BM 13.177), daltroban (BM 13.505), SQ 29548, and AH 23848 (Fig. 1). Each of these agents has been reported to antagonize the platelet aggregatory and vasoconstrictor effects of TXA_2 or a TX mimetic.[3] TX receptor antagonists are equally effective in blocking the contractile and platelet aggregatory effects of TXA_2 and the prostaglandin endoperoxides.

BM 13.177

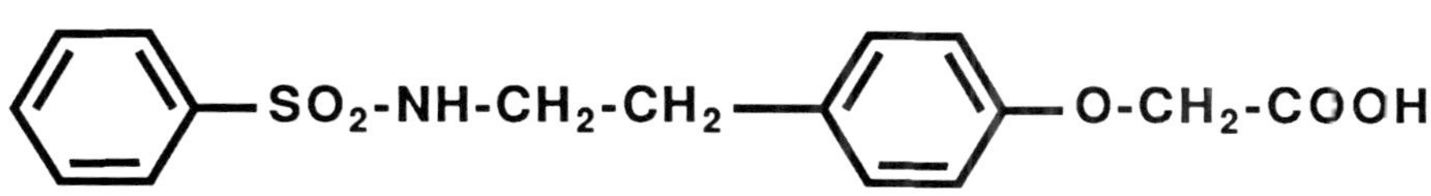

BM 13.505

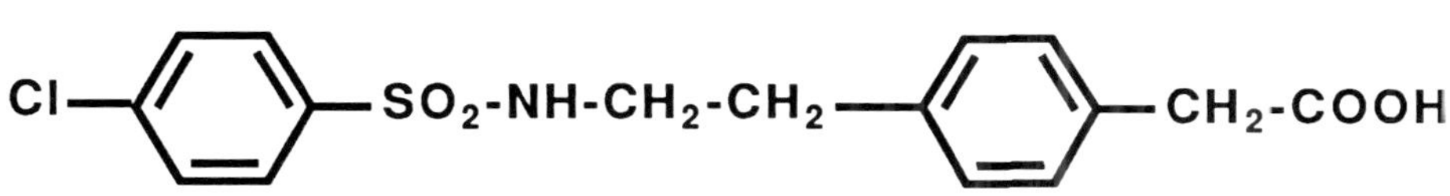

Figure 1 *Structure of the TX receptor antagonists BM 13.177 (sulotroban) and BM 13.505 (daltroban)*

Pathophysiology of TXA_2

In order to implicate TX as a mediator of various cardiovascular pathophysiologic conditions, certain fundamental criteria should be satisfied. First, the formation of a putative mediator such as TXA_2 must be increased in the pathophysiologic condition. Second, the formation of TXA_2 should be temporally and quantitatively correlated with the disease. Third, administration of TX agonists should produce responses that partially mimic the disease. Finally, inhibition of the synthesis, or antagonism of the action of TXA_2, should attenuate the pathophysiologic events. At present, there is considerable evidence, derived predominantly from studies in experimental animals, that TXA_2 is indeed a mediator of certain cardiovascular diseases. Among the cardiovascular disorders in which TXA_2 has been implicated are sudden coronary death, coronary artery thrombosis, and myocardial infarction with reperfusion injury. The involvement of TXA_2 in these pathophysiologic conditions, as well as the possible therapeutic benefits to be derived from the use of a TX receptor antagonist, will be discussed.

Sudden coronary death

Administration of a TX agonist-mimetic, such as U 44619 or carbocyclic TXA_2, or arachidonic acid which is subsequently converted to TXA_2, produces sudden death in anesthetized rats or rabbits. The mechanism of sudden death appears to be due to myocardial ischemia, and pulmonary and cerebral thrombosis. This model of thrombotic sudden death in small animals provides a suitable means for studying the antiplatelet effects of TX receptor antagonists *in vivo*. Figure 2 shows the typical response to the intravenous injection of U 46619 in an anesthetized rat.[5] Approximately 1 min following the injection of U 46619, there is an increase in arterial blood pressure of 20–30 mmHg, and within 2 min, cardiac arrhythmias appear. Finally,

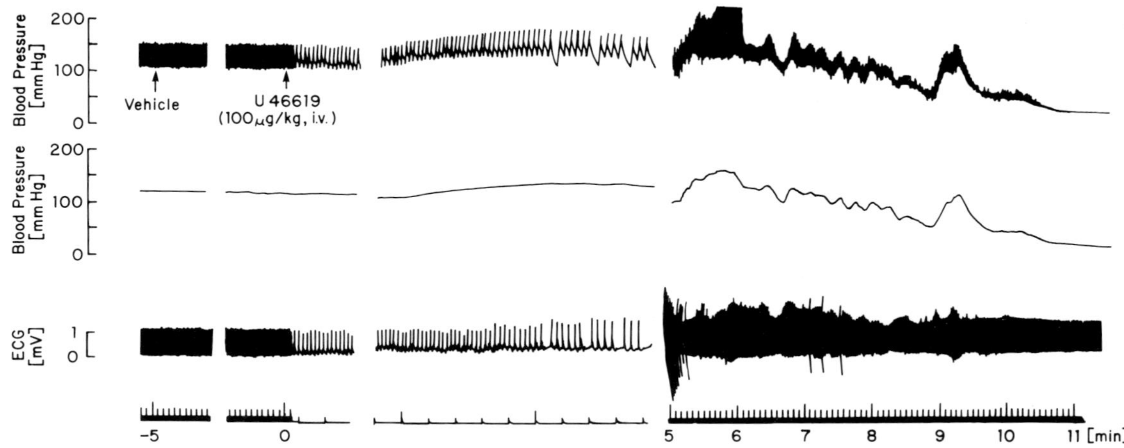

Figure 2 *U 46619-induced sudden death in rat. Upper panel: pulsatile arterial blood pressure; middle panel: mean arterial blood pressure; lower panel: ECG. Death occurred within 11 min of injecting U 46619 (100 μg/kg, i.v.).*

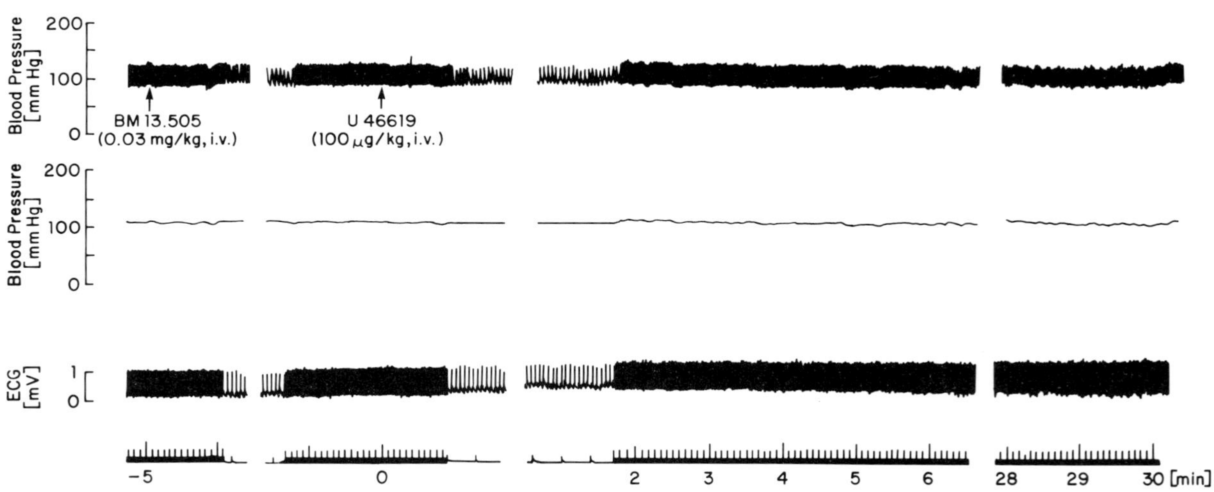

Figure 3 *Prevention of U 46619-induced sudden death in the rat with the thromboxane receptor antagonist daltroban (BM 13.505). For details, see legend to Figure 2. Administration of daltroban (BM 13.505) 5 min prior to the injection of U 46619 prevented sudden death.*

death occurs within 5–15 min as the result of thrombosis. Pretreatment with TX receptor antagonists, such as sulotroban or daltroban, blocks the effects of TXA_2 and prostaglandin endoperoxides (Figure 3). Darius and Lefer [6] reported that a TX synthase inhibitor, dazoxiben, did not block the lethal effects of U 46619, suggesting that TX synthase inhibitors may not prove efficacious when the levels of prostaglandin endoperoxides are sufficiently elevated to activate TX receptors. Thus, TX receptor antagonists may prove to be more effective than TX synthase inhibitors since the effects of the prostaglandin endoperoxides are not blocked by the latter.

Coronary artery thrombosis

Because of its potent effects on platelet function, TXA_2 may be an important mediator of thrombosis in diseased coronary vessels, thereby resulting in myocardial ischemia. It has been demonstrated that coronary artery thrombosis in stenotic canine coronary arteries can be prevented with a TX synthase inhibitor, suggesting that platelet TX formation is an important mediator of this event.[7,8] Ashton *et al.*[9] first reported that a TX receptor antagonist, SQ 29548, reduced the frequency of coronary thrombotic events in a canine model of coronary artery thrombosis. These results with a TX receptor antagonist suggested that the beneficial effects were due directly to blocking the effects of TXA_2, and not secondary to alterations in PGI_2 formation. Bush and Smith[10] and Van der Giessen *et al.*[11] confirmed the anti-thrombotic effects of selective TX receptor blockade with sulotroban in canine and porcine models of coronary artery thrombosis. These and other results provide consistent evidence that agents with higher selectivity than aspirin, such as TX receptor antagonists and TX synthase inhibitors, reduce or eliminate acute episodes of platelet-dependent coronary thrombosis. Interestingly, Fitzgerald *et al.*[12] have recently reported that aspirin was ineffective in reducing coronary artery thrombosis in stenotic canine coronary arteries, yet demonstrated convincingly a reduction in coronary artery thrombosis by a TX receptor antagonist and a TX synthase inhibitor. Moreover, aspirin reversed the antithrombotic effects of the TX receptor antagonist and TX synthase inhibitor. Thus, aspirin-like drugs may not only prove less effective than TX synthase inhibitors or TX receptor antagonists for reducing platelet mediated coronary thrombosis, but may also reverse any protective effects likely to be achieved with the more selective inhibitors of TX.

Coronary fibrinolysis

While the role of TXA_2 in the process of thrombosis has been studied for some time,[7,13] the role of TXA_2 in thrombolysis has only recently been studied. Numerous clinical studies have established the thrombolytic effectiveness of t-PA or streptokinase for recanalization of occluded coronary arteries. However, the reocclusion rate of successfully recanalized blood vessels has been reported to be as high as 45% in patients receiving t-PA. We have recently conducted studies to investigate the mechanism of vascular reocclusion following thrombolysis.[14] These studies demonstrated that at thrombolytic doses, both t-PA and streptokinase induce *ex vivo* platelet hyperaggregability to collagen, arachidonic acid and adenosine diphosphate. Moreover, the anti-aggregatory effect of prostacyclin was reduced by thrombolytic doses of t-PA.[15] The results of these studies suggest that platelet activation which occurs as a consequence of thrombolytic therapy may serve to limit the response to such therapy, and thereby result in unacceptable rates of reocclusion. If, in fact, the thrombolytic agents utilized to achieve recanalization of an occluded coronary vessel also induce a state of platelet activation, the administration of an anti-platelet drug, such as a TX receptor antagonist, would be warranted.

In support of the notion that enhanced TX formation serves to limit the efficacy of fibrinolytic agents, recent investigations in experimental animals have shown TX synthase inhibitors to be useful in enhancing the efficacy of fibrinolytic agents. Mickelson *et al.*[16] reported in a canine model of coronary thrombosis that a TX synthase inhibitor, CGS 13080, was effective in improving coronary blood flow and reducing the incidence of reocclusion from 80% to 20% after coronary thrombolysis with streptokinase. Other studies have examined the benefit of TX receptor blockade for enhancing the thrombolytic efficacy of streptokinase. These studies were conducted with a minimally effective thrombolytic dose of streptokinase in order to assess more accurately the contribution of platelet activation during fibrinolytic therapy. Following thrombus formation in the left circumflex coronary artery of the dog, animals were treated with streptokinase, sulotroban, aspirin, or a combination of streptokinase + sulotroban or streptokinase + aspirin (Table 1). Sulotroban or aspirin had no thrombolytic effect when administered alone, and of 14 animals receiving a low dose of streptokinase, only two reperfused, confirming that the dose of streptokinase used was subthreshold.[17] However, concomitant administration of sulotroban with streptokinase improved the thrombolytic efficacy of streptokinase from 14% to 90%. The use of aspirin in conjunction with streptokinase was significantly less effective. Shebuski *et al.*[18] have also examined the thrombolytic efficacy of sulotroban when used in conjunction with tissue plasminogen activator (t-PA), and found that the TX receptor antagonist decreased the time to clot lysis and reduced the incidence of transient or permanent reocclusion episodes in the dog (Table 2). These data suggest that in addition to the proaggregatory role of TXA_2 in the initiation of coronary artery thrombosis, TXA_2 may also play an important role in limiting the efficacy of thrombolytic agents.

Table 1 *Thrombolytic efficacy of streptokinase, or streptokinase in combination with sulotroban or aspirin in a canine model of stenotic coronary thrombosis*

Group	*Total no. of animals*	*Animals that reperfused*	*Time to reperfusion (min)*
Sulotroban	6	0 (0%)	–
Aspirin	6	0 (0%)	–
Streptokinase	14	2 (14%)	–
Sulotroban + streptokinase	16	14 (88%)[1]	93 ± 10
$Aspirin_1$ + streptokinase	11	2 (18%)[2]	–
$Aspirin_5$ + streptokinase	11	5 (45%)[2]	107 ± 15

[1]$p < 0.05$, compared with the Streptokinase group.

[2]$p < 0.05$, compared to the Sulotroban + Streptokinase group.

Sulotroban (5 mg/kg + 5 mg/kg/hr); Aspirin (1 or 5 mg/kg); Streptokinase (20,000 IU + 2000 IU/min).

Table 2 *Effect of sulotroban on the fibrinolytic efficacy of t-PA in a canine model of stenotic coronary thrombosis*

Group	No.	Time to occlusion (min)	Time to reperfusion (min)	Incidence of reocclusion
t-PA + vehicle	24	41± 5	32± 5	20/24 (83%)
t-PA + sulotroban 1 mg/kg + 1 mg/kg/hr	10	62±17	21± 7	5/10 (50%)
t-PA + sulotroban 10 mg/kg + 10 mg/kg/hr	11	32± 6	11± 2[1]	1/9 (11%)[1]

[1]$p < 0.05$, compared with the t-PA + vehicle group. Two animals in the high dose sulotroban group fibrillated after effective thrombolysis.

Table 3 *Thrombolytic efficacy of streptokinase, in combination with sulotroban or heparin, or in combination with sulotroban + heparin in a canine model of stenotic coronary thrombosis*

Group	Total no. of animals	Animals that reperfused	Time to reperfusion (min)
Sulotroban	6	0 (0%)	-
Streptokinase	10	1 (10%)	-
Sulotroban + Streptokinase	10	9 (90%)[1]	79 ± 11
Heparin + Streptokinase	9	8 (89%)[1]	66 ± 9
Sulotroban + Heparin + Streptokinase	9	9 (100%)[1]	25 ± 5[2]

[1]$p < 0.05$, compared with the Streptokinase group.
[2]$p < 0.05$, compared to the Sulotroban + Streptokinase and Heparin + Streptokinase group. Streptokinase (20,000 IU + 2000 IU/min); Sulotroban (5 mg/kg + 5 mg/kg/hr); Heparin (300 IU/kg + 100 IU/kg/hr).

In a similar canine model of coronary artery thrombosis, the addition of sulotroban to a combination of streptokinase + heparin resulted in a marked reduction in the time to reperfusion (Table 3; cf. ref. 19). More importantly, however, these provocative studies in animal models of coronary artery thrombosis have been confirmed clinically in a study in which sulotroban was administered in conjunction with streptokinase and was found to decrease the time to clot lysis in patients with acute myocardial infarction (Fig. 4). These results suggest that platelet aggregation and fibrin deposition are ongoing processes at the site of an occlusive thrombus, such that antagonism of TXA_2 receptors and inhibition of fibrin formation during thrombolysis may be a valuable means to enhance the efficacy of thrombolytic agents.

Myocardial infarction

The biological activities of TXA_2, including vasoconstriction, platelet aggregation, membrane cytolytic effects and neutrophil adhesion, would be expected to exert a deleterious effect in the setting of myocardial ischemia and reperfusion. Increases in the plasma concentrations of TXB_2 have been measured in animals and humans early after the onset of myocardial ischemia.[20,21] Administration of TXA_2 or a TXA_2 mimetic exacerbates or produces infarcted myocardial tissue.[22] Additionally, selected inhibition of TX formation with a TX synthase inhibitor,[21] as opposed to cyclooxygenase inhibition,[23, 24] is reported to reduce the extent of ischemic myocardial injury. Therefore, TX levels are increased following an episode of myocardial ischemia, and selective inhibition of TX formation is associated with a cardioprotective effect, supporting the notion for the involvement of TXA_2 as a pathological mediator of myocardial infarction.

Recently, the effects of potent and selective TX receptor antagonists on the extent of myocardial reperfusion injury have been investigated. Grover and Schumacher[23, 25] reported that two different TX receptor antagonists, SQ 29548 and SQ 30741, at doses that antagonized the vasoconstrictor effects of a TX mimetic, reduced myocardial reperfusion injury in the dog. A structurally related, but pharmacologically inactive compound, SQ 28585, had no effect on the extent of myocardial injury. Figure 5 shows the effect of another TX receptor antagonist, daltroban (BM 13.505), on myocardial infarct size.[26] Daltroban, at a dose sufficient to block completely the effects of the TX mimetic, U 46619, in the rat,[5] reduced myocardial reperfusion injury. The effects of daltroban were dose dependent since a dose of 3 mg/kg did not provide protection. Furthermore, it was noted that the accumulation of inflammatory cells, specifically neutrophils, were reduced in conjunction to the reduction in myocardial reperfusion injury. The observation that two structurally dissimilar TX receptor antagonists reduced myocardial reperfusion injury, and that the cardioprotective effects were dose-dependent and not shared by a structurally-related but pharmacologically inactive agent, provides convincing evidence that the cardioprotective effects are the result of specific TX receptor antagonism.

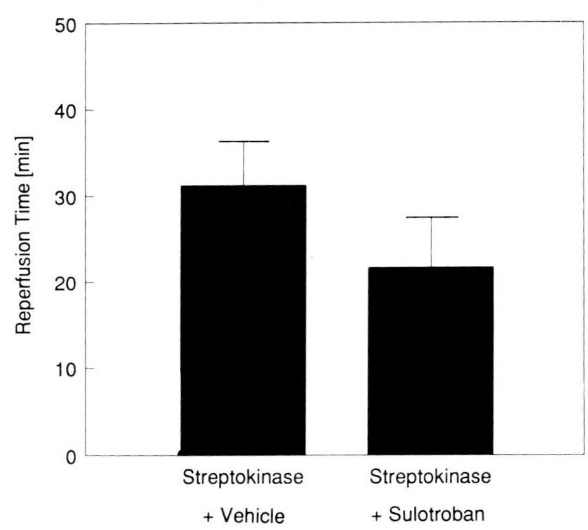

Figure 4 *Effect of the combination of sulotroban + streptokinase vs. streptokinase on the time to reperfusion in patients with an obstructed coronary artery.*

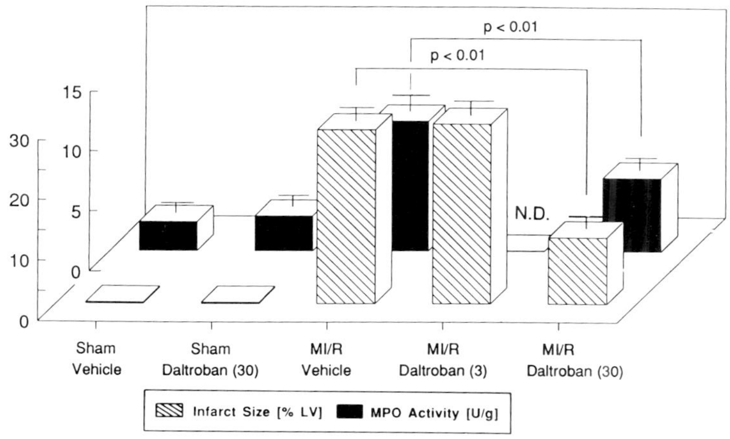

Figure 5 *Reduction of myocardial infarct size in rats subjected to 30 min coronary artery occlusion and 24 hr of reperfusion. Daltroban (BM 13.505) was administered at a dose of 3 or 30 mg/kg, intraperitoneally, 1 min prior to coronary artery occlusion. The extent of neutrophil accumulation in the left ventricular myocardium was determined by measuring the activity of the neutrophil marker enzyme myeloperoxidase (MPO).*

In contrast to the cardioprotective observed with the TX receptor antagonists, cyclooxygenase inhibitors such as aspirin or indomethacin do not provide any direct benefit to the ischemic and reperfused myocardium. Ogletree and Lefer[24] and Grover and Schumacher[23] were unable to demonstrate a cardioprotective effect with aspirin or indomethacin. Although the explanation for the difference between TX receptor antagonists and cyclooxygenase inhibitors is not known at this time, it could be explained by the inhibition of prostacyclin formation by cyclooxygenase inhibitors, thereby preventing the formation of a substance that has been demonstrated to actually protect the myocardium from ischemic insults.

Summary

A number of reports indicate that TX receptor antagonists may be useful in preventing coronary artery reocclusion following fibrinolytic therapy, reducing myocardial ischemia/reperfusion injury and consequent neutrophil accumulation, and preventing thromboembolic sudden death. In fact, TX receptor antagonists may provide greater efficacy than the cyclooxygenase inhibitors, such as aspirin and indomethacin, which do not reduce the incidence of coronary thrombosis, are ineffective in enhancing the fibrinolytic effects of tissue plasminogen activator, and rather than reducing myocardial ischemia/reperfusion injury, may tend to exacerbate the extent of cellular damage. Clinical studies have recently been initiated with a number of different TX receptor antagonists, and adverse clinical effects associated with specific TX receptor blockade are uncommon. Further clinical studies will be required to confirm the provocative animal studies outlined herein, as well as defining the precise role of TX as a mediator of coronary vasospasm, coronary thrombosis and myocardial reperfusion injury in humans.

Address for correspondence: Dr. Edward F. Smith III, SmithKline Beecham Pharmaceuticals, plc Department of Pharmacology, P.O.B. 1539 (L-510), King of Prussia, PA 19406, U.S.A.

References

1. Smith E F III, Rucker W, Schror K, RCS from human platelets: is it only thromboxane?

Europ. J. Pharmacol. 95, 1983, 121–124.
2. Verheggen R, Schror K, The modification of platelet-induced coronary vasoconstriction by a thromboxane receptor antagonist. *J. Cardiovasc. Pharmacol. 8*, 1986, 483–490.
3. Bush L R, Smith S G, Antagonism of U-46619-induced aggregation of human and canine platelets by four TxA_2 receptor antagonists. *Thromb. Res. 44*, 1986, 337–341.
4. Mais D E, DeHoll D, Sightler H, Halushka P V, Different pharmacologic activities for 13-azapinane thromboxane A_2 analogs in platelets and blood vessels. *Europ. J. Pharmacol. 148*, 1988, 309–315.
5. Smith E F III, McDonald J, Protective effects of the thromboxane receptor antagonists BM 13.177 and BM 13.505 against U 46619-induced sudden death in rats. *Pharmacology 36*, 1988, 340–347.
6. Darius H, Lefer A M, Antiaggregatory effects of thromboxane receptor antagonist *in vivo*. *Thromb. Res. 40*, 1985, 663–675.
7. Aiken J W, Pharmacology of thromboxane synthetase inhibitors. In *Advances in Prostaglandin, Thromboxane and Leukotriene Research,* Vol 11, Samuelsson B, Paoletti R and Ramwell P (eds), Raven Press, New York, 1983, pp 253–258.
8. Bush L R, Campbell W B, Buja L M, Tilton G D, Willerson J T, Effects of the selective thromboxane synthetase inhibitor dazoxiben on variations in cyclic blood flow in stenosed canine coronary arteries. *Circulation 69*, 1984, 1161–1170.
9. Ashton J H, Schmitz J M, Campbell W B, Ogletree M L, Raheja S, Taylor A L, Fitzgerald C, Buja L M, Willerson J T, Inhibition of cyclic flow variations in stenosed canine coronary arteries by thromboxane A_2/prostaglandin H_2 receptor antagonists. *Circ. Res. 59*, 1986, 568–578.
10. Bush L R, Smith S G, Comparative and combined effects of U-63557A, a TxA_2 synthetase inhibitor, and BM 13.177, a TxA_2 receptor antagonist, on cyclic flow reductions in stenosed canine coronary arteries. *Fed. Proc.46*, 1987, 1316.
11. Van der Giessen W J, Zijlstra F J, Berk L, Verdouw P D, The effect of the thromboxane receptor antagonist BM 13.177 on experimentally induced coronary artery thrombosis in the pig. *Europ. J. Pharmacol. 147*, 1988, 241–248.
12. Fitzgerald D J, Fragetta J, FitzGerald G A, Prostaglandin endoperoxides modulate the response to thromboxane synthase inhibition during coronary thrombosis. *J. Clin. Invest. 82*, 1988, 1708–1713.
13. Simpson P J, Smith C B, Rosenthal G, Lucchesi B R, Reduction in the incidence of thrombosis by the thromboxane synthase inhibitor CGS 13080 in a canine model of coronary artery injury. *J. Pharmacol. Exper. Therap. 238*, 1986, 497–501.
14. Ohlstein E H, Storer B, Fujita T, Shebuski R J, Tissue-type plasminogen activator and streptokinase induce platelet hyperaggregability in the rabbit. *Thromb. Res. 46*, 1987, 575–585.
15. Shebuski R J, Ohlstein E H, Attenuation of platelet responsiveness to prostacyclin (PGI_2) after tissue-type plasminogen activator (t-PA). *Circulation 76*, 1987, IV–338.
16. Mickelson J K, Simpson P J, Gallas M T, Lucchesi B R (1987). Thromboxane synthetase inhibition with CGS 13080 improves coronary blood flow after streptokinase-induced thrombolysis. *Am. Heart J. 113*, 1987, 1345–1352.
17. Kopia G A, Kopaciewicz L J, Ohlstein E H, Comparison of the thrombolytic efficacy of streptokinase in combination with the thromboxane receptor antagonist, sulotroban, or aspirin. *FASEB J. 3*, 1989, A1208.
18. Shebuski R J, Smith J M Jr, Storer B L, Granett J R, Bugelski P J, Influence of selective endoperoxide/thromboxane A_2 receptor antagonism with sulotroban on lysis time and reocclusion rate after tissue plasminogen activator-induced coronary thrombolysis in the dog.

J. Pharmacol. Exper. Therap. 246, 1988, 790–796.

19. Kopia G A, Kopaciewicz L J, Ohlstein E H, Horohonich S, Storer B L, Shebuski R J, Combination of the thromboxane receptor antagonist, sulotroban (BM 13.177, SK&F 95587), with streptokinase: demonstration of thrombolytic synergy. *J. Pharmacol. Exper. Therap. 250*, 1989, 887–895.
20. Lewy R I, Smith J B, Silver M J, Saia J, Walinsky P, Wiener L, Detection of thromboxane B_2 in peripheral blood of patients with Prinzmetal's angina. *Prostaglandins Med. 5*, 1979, 243–248.
21. Smith E F III, Lefer A M, Smith J B, Influence of thromboxane inhibition on the severity of myocardial ischemia in cats. *Canad. J. Physiol. Pharmacol. 58*, 1980, 294–300.
22. Smith E F III, Lefer A M, Arahony D, Smith J B, Magolda R L, Claremon D, Nicolaou K C, Carbocyclic thromboxane A_2: aggravation of myocardial ischemia by a new synthetic thromboxane analog. *Prostaglandins 21*, 1981, 443–456.
23. Grover G J, Schumacher W A, Effect of the thromboxane receptor antagonist SQ 30, 741 on ultimate infarct size, reperfusion injury and coronary flow reserve. *J. Pharmacol. Exptl. Therap. 248*, 1989, 484–491.
24. Ogletree M L, Lefer A M, Influence of nonsteroidal anti-inflammatory agents on myocardial ischemia in the cat. *J. Pharmacol. Exper. Therap. 197*, 1976, 582–593.
25. Grover G J, Schumacher W A, Effect of the thromboxane receptor antagonist SQ 29,548 on myocardial infarct size in dogs. *J. Cardiovasc. Pharmacol. 11*, 1988, 29–35.
26. Smith E F III, Griswold D E, Egan J W, Hillegass L M, DiMartino M J, Reduction of myocardial damage and polymorphonuclear leukocyte accumulation following coronary artery occlusion and reperfusion by the thromboxane receptor antagonist BM 13.505. *J. Cardiovasc. Pharmacol. 13*, 1989, 715–722.

Chapter 12

NEW DEVELOPMENTS IN THROMBOLYTIC THERAPY

D. Collen

University of Leuven, Belgium, and

H. K. Gold

Harvard Medical School, Boston, MA, USA

Summary

Thrombotic complications of cardiovascular disease are principal causes of death and disability and, consequently, thrombolysis could favorably influence the outcome of such life-threatening diseases as myocardial infarction, cerebrovascular thrombosis and venous thromboembolism.

Thrombolytic agents are plasminogen activators that convert plasminogen, the inactive proenzyme of the fibrinolytic system in blood, to the proteolytic enzyme plasmin. Plasmin dissolves the fibrin of a blood clot, but may also degrade normal components of the hemostatic system and predispose to bleeding. Currently, five thrombolytic agents are either approved for clinical use or under clinical investigation in patients with acute myocardial infarction. These include streptokinase, urokinase, recombinant tissue-type plasminogen activator (rt-PA), anisoylated plasminogen streptokinase activator complex (anistreplase) and single chain urokinase-type plasminogen activator (scu-PA, prourokinase). The first generation thrombolytic agents, streptokinase (and probably also urokinase), are only moderately efficacious and their administration is associated with extensive systemic fibrinogen breakdown. In comparative studies performed in patients with acute myocardial infarction, recombinant tissue-type plasminogen activator (rt-PA) is a more effective and fibrin-specific thrombolytic agent than streptokinase. The acylated plasminogen streptokinase activator complex (anistreplase) has a profile of thrombolytic efficacy and fibrin-specificity that is similar or somewhat better than that of streptokinase, but has the advantage that it can be administered by bolus injection. Single chain urokinase-type plasminogen activator is more fibrin-specific than urokinase. Comparative data on the efficacy and safety of this agent are limited as it is in the early stage of clinical investigation.

Reduction of infarct size, preservation of ventricular function and/or reduction in mortality have been observed with streptokinase, rt-PA and anistreplase. Therefore, thrombolytic therapy will probably become routine therapy for early acute myocardial infarction.

In patients with acute myocardial infarction, intravenous streptokinase recanalizes 40–45% of occluded coronary arteries and reduces mortality by 25%; it costs approximately $200 for a therapeutic dose of 1,500,000 units. Recombinant tissue-type plasminogen activator (rt-PA) is more potent for coronary arterial thrombolysis, producing both more rapid and more frequent (65–70%) reperfusion, but it costs over $1000 for a therapeutic dose of 100 mg. Side effects (mainly bleeding) and the incidence of reocclusion associated with the use of streptokinase and rt-PA are not markedly different. Whether the higher efficacy of rt-PA will translate into a comparably larger reduction of mortality remains to be determined in large comparative clinical trials. Both agents are available for clinical use. The choice of agent for the treatment of acute myocardial infarction at present must be based on considerations of lower cost of streptokinase versus the higher efficacy for coronary recanalization of rt-PA.

Recent reviews of thrombolytic agents have reached apparently contradictory conclusions with respect to the comparative properties of thrombolytic agents.[1-3] In particular, the data on the relative efficacy for coronary thrombolysis, the speed of reperfusion, the frequency of reocclusion, the occurrence of bleeding complications, and the impact on mortality have been presented and interpreted differently.

All available thrombolytic agents still suffer significant shortcomings, including the need for large doses in order to be therapeutically efficient, and limited fibrin-specificity with residual toxicity in terms of bleeding complications. New developments towards greater efficacy and fibrin-specificity of thrombolytic therapy include the use of combinations of synergistic thrombolytic agents, mutants of t-PA and scu-PA, chimeric t-PA/scu-PA molecules, antibody-targeted thrombolytic agents, and/or combinations of fibrin-dissolving agents with anti-platelet strategies.

In this communication, we will briefly review the components of the fibrinolytic system, the mechanism of fibrin-specific thrombolysis, the present state of clinical trials with thrombolytic agents in acute myocardial infarction, and finally, new trends in thrombolytic therapy.

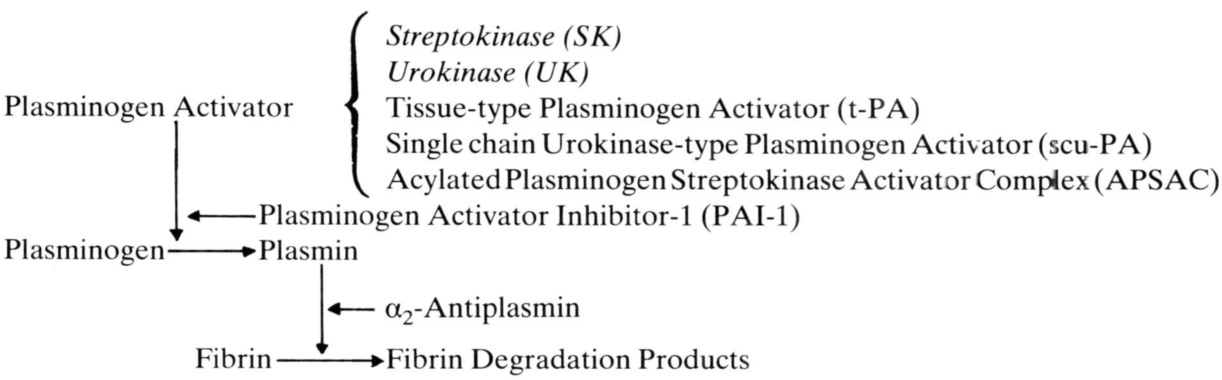

Figure 1 *Schematic representation of the fibrinolytic system*

The fibrinolytic system

Components of the fibrinolytic system

The fibrinolytic system, schematically represented in Figure 1, contains a proenzyme, plasminogen, which can be converted to the active enzyme plasmin by the action of several different types of plasminogen activators. Plasmin is a serine protease that digests fibrin to soluble degradation products. Natural inhibition of the fibrinolytic system occurs both at the level of the plasminogen activator and at the level of plasmin.[4-6]

Plasminogen is a single chain glycoprotein consisting of 790 amino acids that is converted to plasmin by cleavage of the Arg560–Val561 peptide bond. The plasminogen molecule contains structures, called lysine binding sites, which mediate its binding to fibrin and accelerate the interaction between plasmin and its physiological inhibitor, α_2-antiplasmin. The lysine binding sites play a crucial role in the regulation of fibrinolysis. Plasminogen binds to platelets and endothelial cells, and this binding enhances the conversion to plasmin.

Plasminogen activators are serine proteases with a high specificity for plasminogen. The hydrolysis of the Arg560–Val561 peptide bond of plasminogen yields the active enzyme, plasmin.

Streptokinase is a nonenzyme protein with molecular weight of 47,000 that is produced by beta-hemolytic streptococci. Streptokinase activates the fibrinolytic system indirectly by forming a 1:1 stoichiometric complex with plasminogen. The formation of this complex exposes an active site in the modified plasminogen moiety, whereby the complex becomes a potent plasminogen activator.

Anistreplase (anisoylated plasminogen streptokinase activator complex) is an inactive derivative of the plasminogen-streptokinase activator complex obtained by acylation of its active site serine. Spontaneous deacylation at physiological pH with a t1/2 of 35 to 70 min promotes its reactivation.

Urokinase is a trypsin-like serine protease composed of two polypeptide chains, connected by a disulfide bridge, which activates plasminogen directly to plasmin. Single chain urokinase-type plasminogen activator (scu-PA) or pro-urokinase is a single chain glycoprotein containing 411 amino acids, which is converted to urokinase by hydrolysis of the Lys158–Ile159 peptide bond.

scu-PA has very little activity towards low molecular weight substrates *in vitro* but does possess intrinsic plasminogen activating potential. The catalytic efficiency of scu-PA is approximately two orders of magnitude lower than that of urokinase.

Tissue-type plasminogen activator (t-PA) is a trypsin-like serine protease composed of 527 amino acids. It occurs either as a single chain glycoprotein or as a two chain proteolytic derivative, but both forms have comparable enzymatic properties.

t-PA is a poor plasminogen activator in the absence of fibrin, but it binds specifically to fibrin and activates plasminogen at the fibrin surface several hundred-fold more efficiently than in the circulation.

t-PA binds to endothelial cells and is cleared through a saturable, probably hepatic mechanism.

α_2-antiplasmin is a glycoprotein of the serine protease inhibitor (Serpin) superfamily, composed of 452 amino acids with Arg364-Met365 as the reactive site. α_2-antiplasmin reacts very rapidly with plasmin, first to form a reversible but inactive complex, which is then slowly converted into an irreversible complex. The rapidity of the first step of the reaction is dependent on the presence of free lysine binding sites and a free active center in the plasmin molecule.

Plasminogen activator inhibitor-1 (PAI-1) is a fast acting inhibitor of t-PA and urokinase occurring at very low concentration in the blood, but which may be significantly increased in several disease states including venous thromboembolism and ischemic heart disease. It is a Serpin, composed of 379 amino acids with Arg346-Met347 as the reactive site.

Mechanism of fibrin-specific thrombolysis

Plasmin, the proteolytic enzyme of the fibrinolytic system has a low substrate specificity. In purified systems it will degrade fibrinogen almost as well as fibrin and, when circulating freely in the blood, it will degrade a number of plasma proteins including fibrinogen and the blood coagulation factors V and VIII. Plasmin generated in blood will, however, rapidly be neutralized by α_2-antiplasmin via the mechanism detailed above. Extensive systemic activation of the fibrinolytic system will result in α_2-antiplasmin depletion, excess free plasmin generation, and secondary hemostatic breakdown. In contrast, plasmin that is generated at the fibrin surface has both its lysine binding sites and active center occupied and thus is only very slowly inactivated by α_2-antiplasmin.[4]

Clot-specific thrombolysis will, in view of these interactions, require plasminogen activation at, or in the vicinity of, the fibrin clot. The two physiological plasminogen activators, t-PA and scu-PA, exert clot-specificity in a plasma environment via entirely different molecular mechanisms.[5] t-PA is relatively, but not totally, inactive in the absence of fibrin. It binds specifically to fibrin, thereafter acquiring a high affinity for plasminogen, resulting in preferential plasminogen activation on the fibrin clot. In a plasma milieu, relatively fibrin-specific clot lysis can be obtained within a rather narrow concentration range with scu-PA. In the absence of fibrin, no significant plasminogen activation occurs. Apparently, plasma exerts a competitive inhibitory effect that is reversed by fibrin.[5] In addition, fibrin-bound plasminogen may be more sensitive to activation by scu-PA and scu-PA may be converted to the more active urokinase at the clot surface.[6]

Thrombolytic therapy in acute myocardial infarction

In the late 1970s, it was recognized that thrombosis within the infarct related coronary artery played a major role in the pathogenesis of acute myocardial infarction.[7] It was further recognized that early administration of either intracoronary or intravenous streptokinase resulted in reperfusion of 75 and 45% of patients, respectively.[8] This has formed the basis for several large scale studies employing intravenous thrombolytics with the intention to 1) define the real impact of early coronary artery reperfusion on patient survival and 2) establish patterns of efficacy and safety for new and potentially improved thrombolytic agents. The agents used for thrombolytic therapy in humans can be classified in two main categories: (a) the 'classical' thrombolytic agents, streptokinase and urokinase, and (b) the 'second-generation' thrombolytic agents, t-PA, scu-PA, and acylated plasminogen streptokinase activator complex (anistreplase).

Placebo-controlled trials with mortality end-points

The results of the major placebo-controlled clinical studies with intravenous thrombolytic therapy in patients with acute myocardial infarction are shown in Table 1.

Streptokinase

The first major study employing intravenous streptokinase in early acute myocardial infarction and demonstrating relative improvement in survival was carried out in 11,806 patients and reported as the GISSI Study.[9,10] Life-threatening bleeding was observed in only 0.3% of patients receiving streptokinase and judged not to be a limitation for therapy. This study confirmed and extended the observations with intracoronary streptokinase.[11] The positive results of the GISSI trial were not confirmed in a very similar but somewhat smaller study of the ISAM study group.[12] Furthermore, in the ISAM-study, life-threatening bleeding was more common, occurring in 0.8% of patients. However, the ISIS-2 study has confirmed and extended the GISSI findings in 17,189 patients with an in-hospital mortality reduction from 11.7 to 8.9% in patients receiving streptokinase.[13] This study also showed a significant reduction of mortality with aspirin and that the effects of streptokinase and aspirin are additive. Two additional studies[14,15] have provided further evidence of the effect of streptokinase therapy on mortality reduction and on its relative safety.

In aggregate, these studies are suggestive of two conclusions. First, the intravenous administration of streptokinase early (preferably within 4 hours) in acute myocardial infarction

Table 1 *Major placebo-controlled clinical trials with intravenous thrombolytic therapy in acute myocardial infarction*

Study	*Patient number*	*Adjunctive Therapy*		*Major Bleeding(%)*		*Neurological Event Rate (%)*			*Early Mortality Rate (%)*			*p*
		Aspirin	*Heparin*	*Placebo*	*Active*	*Definition*	*Placebo*	*Active*	*Endpoint*	*Placebo*	*Active*	
A. Streptokinase												
GISSI[9,10]	11,806	14%	21%	?	0.3	Stroke	0.9	1.1	21d	13.0	10.7	0.0002
						SK-CVA		0.2				
ISAM[12]	1,741	+	+	?	0.8	ICB	0	0.5	21d	7.1	6.3	NS
W. Wash[14]	368	?	+	(0.7)	(13)	ICB	0	0.5	14d	9.7	6.3	NS
N. Zealand[15]	219	+	+	0	1	ICB	0	0	30d	12.9	2.5	0.012
ISIS-2[13]	17,189	+/−	−	0.2	0.6	Stroke	0.9	0.8	35d	11.7	8.9	0.0001
						SK-ICB		0.1–0.2				
B. rt-PA												
ECSG[19]	721	+	+	1.9	3.7	Stroke	0.5	2.0	14d	5.7	2.8	0.053
						rt-PA-ICB	?	1.4				
ASSET[20]	5,111	−	+(24hr)	0.4	1.4	Stroke	1.0	1.1	30d	9.8	7.2	0.002
C. APSAC												
AIMS[24]	1,004	?	+	?	?	Stroke	1.0	0.4	30d	12.2	6.4	0.0016

Abbreviations. ICB: intracerebral bleeding; CVA: cerebrovascular accident; SK-CVA: CVA associated with streptokinase therapy; SK-ICB: ICB associated with SK therapy; rt-PA-ICB: ICB associated with rt-PA therapy.

is of benefit to both early and late patient survival. Second, the incidence of life-threatening side effects, predominantly major bleeding and intracranial hemorrhage, is not negligible but they occur consistently in less than 1% of the patients treated with streptokinase.

Tissue-type plasminogen activator

Following the demonstration of the potential of natural t-PA as a thrombolytic agent, an intensive effort was launched to enhance its production by recombinant DNA technology.[16] Subsequently, improved left ventricular function[17–19] and reduced mortality[19,20] were demonstrated with recombinant t-PA (rt-PA) in placebo-controlled trials (Table 1).

A major recent concern with the use of rt-PA has been the occurrence of intracerebral bleeding. This complication occurred in 1.6% of 1014 patients who received 150 mg of rt-PA combined with heparin and aspirin.[21] This frequency has been reduced to 0.5% in 1452 patients of the TIMI trial with the use of 100 mg of rt-PA.[21] In the large scale placebo-controlled ASSET trial,[20] the stroke rates in the rt-PA and placebo groups were, however, similar.

Thus, initial evaluation of rt-PA in myocardial infarction has been promising, suggesting its potential role as an improved thrombolytic agent. However, its use is not risk-free despite its relatively higher clot-selectivity than streptokinase.

Acylated plasminogen streptokinase activator complex

In controlled studies comparing intravenous anistreplase with intravenous or intracoronary streptokinase, anistreplase was found to cause reperfusion at a frequency intermediate between that of intravenous and intracoronary streptokinase.[22,23] A marked reduction in mortality was obtained with anistreplase in the AIMS Study.[24]

Comparative biological properties of thrombolytic agents

The relevant biological properties of thrombolytic agents in terms of their benefit/risk ratio in acute myocardial infarction comprise their efficacy for coronary artery recanalization, the speed of reperfusion, the incidence of reocclusion, the frequency and severity of bleeding complications and their effect on mortality.

At present, insufficient results of comparative clinical trials are available to allow definitive quantitative comparison of the relative efficacy and safety of the various thrombolytic agents, although such attempts have recently been made.[3,25] At the present time, sufficient information is available from randomized controlled trials or from uncontrolled trials with comparable endpoints, to allow a semi-quantitative comparison of recombinant t-PA with streptokinase and APSAC with streptokinase. For urokinase and scu-PA, such comparisons can be made only in a preliminary and tentative manner. The comparative properties of thrombolytic agents, to the extent that they can at present be evaluated, are summarized in Table 2, and will be further detailed below.

Efficacy for coronary thrombolysis

The efficacy of plasminogen activators for coronary thrombolysis in patients with acute myocardial infarction has been established by coronary angiography in 'reperfusion' trials, in which patients with occluded coronary arteries, selected by angiography *before* treatment, were subjected to angiography at different time intervals after the start of thrombolytic therapy. Alternatively, 'patency' trials have only studied patients by angiography at different time intervals *after* the start of thrombolytic therapy. Furthermore, coronary thrombolysis, either spontaneous or in association with thrombolytic therapy, is a time-dependent phenomenon. Even without thrombolytic therapy, more than half of the patients with acute myocardial infarction will eventually (i.e. within several days) have a patent infarct-related vessel.[7, 19, 26] The time window after the onset of symptoms within which reperfusion is useful for myocardial salvage is limited to several hours, which reduces the time for relevant comparisons of the efficacy of reperfusion to a couple of hours after the start of the therapy.

Table 2 *Comparative properties of thrombolytic agents in acute myocardial infarction*

	Streptokinase	*APSAC*	*Urokinase*	*scu-PA*	*t-PA*
Coronary thrombolysis					
Reperfusion	+(43%)	+or++	+or++	?	+++(68%)
Patency	+(52%)	++	+or++	++or+++	+++(75%)
Speed of reperfusion	+	+or++	?	+or++	++
Reocclusion	++	+or++	+or++	+or++	++
Fibrin-specificity	–	–	–or+	+	++
Bleeding complications	++	++	?	+or++	+
Strokes	+(1%)*	+	?	–	+or++(?)
Allergic side effects	+	+	–	–	–
Duration of infusion (min)	60	5	30–60	60	180
Dose (currently recommended or most frequently used)	1,500,000 units (~15 mg)	30 mg	3,000,000 units (~30 mg)	70–80 mg	100 mg
Early mortality reduction	+(25%)	+or++	?	?	+or++

At present there is insufficient data from comparative controlled trials with thrombolytic agents to allow definitive quantitative conclusions on their relative properties. In this table an attempt is made to grade relative properties semiquantitatively on the basis of results of controlled trials or of uncontrolled trials with sufficiently comparable design and endpoints. When sufficient data are available, quantitative estimates are included within brackets.

* The stroke rate in the absence of thrombolytic therapy is approximately 1%

Table 3 *Reperfusion demonstrated by coronary angiography at 60–180 minutes after the start of therapy in patients with acute myocardial infarction*

Study	*Dose**	*Mean time to treatment (hrs)*	*Reperfusion (percent)*	*Angiographic endpoint (**)*
A. *Streptokinase*				
Neuhaus *et al.* 1983[27]	1.7M, 60 min	3.7	60 (24/40)	60 min
Schröder *et al.* 1983[28]	0.5 M, 30 min	3.8	52 (11/21)	60 min
Rogers *et al.* 1983 (1983)[29]	1 M, 45 min	6.5	44 (7/16)	75 min
Alderman *et al.* 1984[30]	0.725 M, 85 min	3.4	62 (8/13)	90 min
Spann *et al.* 1984[31]	0.85–1.5 M, 60 min	3.5	49 (21/43)	60 min
Hillis *et al.* 1985[32]	1.5 M, 60 min	4.5	32 (11/34)	90 min
TIMI-I Phase I 1985[33]	1.5 M, 60 min	4.8	31 (37/119)	90 min
de Marneffe *et al.* 1985[34]	1.5 M, 30 min	3.6	80 (8/10)	60 min
Total		4.3	43 (127/296)	
B. *rt-PA*				
Collen *et al.* 1984[35]	TC, 0.5–0.75 mg/kg 30–180 min	4.7	75 (25/33)	90 min
TIMI-1 1985[33]	TC, 50 mg/90 min	4.8	62 (70/113)	90 min
Williams *et al.* 1986[36]	TC, 50 mg/90 min	4.8	68 (25/37)	90 min
Gold *et al.* 1986[37]	TC, 0.4–0.75 mg/kg 60–120 min	3.0	83 (24/29)	60 min
TIMI-B 1987[38]	SC, 70 mg/90 min	4.6	71 (59/83)	90 min
TIMI-C 1987[38]	SC, 100 mg/90 min	4.6	68 (42/62)	90 min
Total		4.4	69 (245/357)	
C. *APSAC*				
Bonnier *et al.* 1987[39]	30 U	2.5	64 (23/36)	90 min
De Wilde *et al.* 1985[40]	30 U	(< 3)	67 (10/15)	90 min
Marder *et al.* 1986[41]	30 U	4.1	60 (9/15)	90 min
Timmis *et al.* 1987[42]	30 U	3.3	53 (8/15)	90 min
Anderson 1988[23]	30 U	(< 6)	51 (59/115)	90 min
Total		56 (109/196)		

*M: mega units; TC: two-chain; SC: single-chain

** Studies with angiography performed many hours or days after therapy have not been included in this analysis

Tables 3 and 4 summarize the results of available efficacy trials with intravenous streptokinase, rt-PA, APSAC and urokinase strictly grouped as 'reperfusion' and 'patency' trials. Only trials with reasonably comparable endpoints, i.e., angiography around 90 minutes (60 to 180 minutes) after the onset of the infusion are included in the analysis. Results of reperfusion trials, with a mean time from onset of symptoms to treatment of more than 4 hours, show a 60% higher efficacy of rt-PA as compared with streptokinase (69 vs 43%), and an intermediate

Table 4 *Patency demonstrated by coronary angiography at 60–180 minutes after the start of therapy in patients with acute myocardial infarction*

Study	*Dose**	*Mean time to treatment (hrs)*	*Reperfusion (percent)*	*Angiographic endpoint* **
A. *Streptokinase*				
Taylor *et al.* 1984 [43]	0.85 M, 60 min	3.2	77 (17/22)	60 min
Schwartz *et al.* 1984 [44]	1.5 M, 90 min	2.5	45 (25/55)	90 min
Verstraete *et al.* 1985 [45]	1.5 M, 60 min	2.6	55 (34/62)	90 min
Cribier *et al.* 1986 [46]	1.5 M, 60 min	3.1	52 (11/21)	60 min
Brochier *et al.* 1987 [22]	1.5 M, 60 min	2.8	56 (24/43)	105 min
Monnier *et al.* 1987 [47]	1.5 M, 60 min	2.5	64 (7/11)	150 min
Chesebro *et al.* 1988 [48]	1.5 M, 60 min	4.7	42 (61/146)	90 min
Stack *et al.* 1988 [49]	1.5 M, 60 min	3.0	44 (95/216)	90 min
Lopez-Sendon *et al.* 1988 [50]	1.5 M, 60 min	2.9	58 (14/24)	90 min
Vogt *et al.* 1988 [66]			72 (21/31)	
PRIMI 1989 [70]	1.5 M, 60 min	< 4	64 (124/194)	90 min
Total		3.0	52 (433/825)	
B. *rt-PA*				
Verstraete *et al.* 1985 [51]	TC, 0.75 mg/kg, 90 min	3.4	61 (38/60)	90 min
Verstraete *et al.* 1985 [45]	TC, 0.75 mg/kg, 90 min	3.0	70 (43/61)	90 min
Verstraete *et al.* 1987 [52]	TC, 40 mg/90 min	2.5	66 (78/119)	90 min
Topol *et al.* 1987 [53]	SC, 1.25 mg/kg, 3 hr	4.0	71 (27/38)	90 min
Topol *et al.* 1987 [54]	SC, 150 mg, 6–8 hr	3.9	75 (288/386)	90 min
Topol *et al.* 1987 [55]	SC, 150 mg, 6–8 hr	3.8	67 (60/89)	90 min
		2.1	81 (43/53)	90 min
Topol *et al.* 1988 [56]	SC, 1.5 mg/kg, 3 hr	2.8	79 (104/132)	90 min
Simoons *et al.* 1988 [57]	SC, 100 mg, 3 hr	2.6	89 (160/180)	90 min
Johns *et al.* 1988 [58]	SC, 1 mg/kg, 90 min	(< 6)	76 (52/68)	90 min
TIMI-IIA 1988 [59]	SC, 100 mg, 90 min	2.8	76 (47/62)	120 min
	SC, 70 mg, 90 min	3.2	75 (97/130)	120 min
McNeill *et al.* 1988 [60]	SC, 100 mg, 90 min	2.3	82 (14/17)	90 min
Neuhaus *et al.* 1988 [61]	SC, 70 mg, 90 min	(< 6)	69 (43/62)	
Heuhaus *et al.* 1988 [62]	SC, 100 mg, 90 min	2.8	86 (30/35)	90 min
Total		3.0	75(1,124/1,492)	
C. *APSAC*				
Kasper *et al.* 1986 [63]	30 U	2.5	84 (42/50)	90 min
Brochier *et al.* 1987 [22]	30 U	(< 6)	72 (28/39)	90 min
Monassier *et al.* 1987 [64]	30 U	(< 6)	74 (37/50)	90 min

Table 4 *Continued*

Study	*Dose**	*Mean time to treatment (hrs)*	*Reperfusion (percent)*	*Angiographic endpoint (**)*
Relik-Van Wely *et al.* 1988 [65]	30 U	(< 4)	76 (75/99)	90 min
Lopéz-Sendón *et al.* 1988 [50]	30 U	2.9	90 (18/20)	90 min
Vogt *et al.* 1988 [66]	30 U	2.6	76 (23/30)	90 min
Total		2.7	77 (223/288)	
D. *Urokinase*				
Mathey *et al.* 1988 [67]	2 M bolus		60 (30/50)	90 min
Neuhaus *et al.* 1988 [68]	1.5 M bolus plus 1.5 M over 90 min		63 (40/63)	90 min
Total			62 (70/113)	

*M: mega units; TC: two-chain; SC: single-chain

** Studies with angiography performed many hours or days after therapy have not been included in this analysis

value for APSAC (56% reperfusion). Patency trials with a mean time from onset of symptoms to treatment of usually less than 3 hours show a 50% higher efficacy for rt-PA (75%) and for APSAC (77%) as compared with streptokinase (52%). The lower frequencies of open arteries in the reperfusion trials as compared with the patency trials (43 vs. 52% for streptokinase, 69 vs 75% for rt-PA and 56 vs 77% for APSAC) may be due either to inclusion of some patients with initially open arteries in the patency trials or to a somewhat higher efficacy of these agents towards fresher coronary clots. In one study, patency rates of 75% at 90 minutes obtained with 1 mg/kg of rt-PA could not be further increased with the combined use of high doses of rt-PA (1 mg/kg over 1 hr) and of urokinase (2,000,000 units)[68] suggesting that a significant proportion of occluded coronary arteries may be refractory to reperfusion with thrombolytic agents and that the maximally obtainable reperfusion frequencies have been approached with rt-PA at the currently recommended dosage.

Two randomized trials have been reported directly comparing the efficacy of streptokinase and rt-PA by angiography 90 minutes after the start of the infusion, namely the TIMI-I trial[33,69] and the first trial of the European Cooperative Study Group (ECSG).[45] The TIMI-I trial was a reperfusion trial, whereas the ECGS trial was a patency trial. However, patency data from the TIMI-I trial have also recently been reported, allowing pooling of the patency results of these two comparative trials.[48] The coronary patency at 90 minutes after the start of the infusion, substratified for patients treated within 3 hours of the onset of symptoms, and for patients treated between 3 and 6 hours, are summarized in Table 5. The patency at 90 minutes was significantly higher in both subgroups of patients treated with rt-PA as compared to patients treated with streptokinase. The overall frequency of patent coronary arteries with rt-PA (143 of 204 patients, 70%) relative to streptokinase (95 of 207 patients, 46%) is 52% higher.

The results summarized in Tables 3 to 5 thus show that, when measured within a time frame useful for salvaging myocardial tissue, streptokinase is a less efficient agent for coronary thrombolysis, reperfusing at best one out of two occluded arteries, whereas rt-PA is significantly more efficient, reperfusing at least two out of three occluded arteries. Thus, the predictions based on the biochemical properties of rt-PA have indeed translated into a higher efficacy for coronary thrombolysis.

Table 5 *Relative efficacy of rt-PA and streptokinase for coronary thrombolysis in patients with acute myocardial infarction: randomized trials*

Time from onset of symptoms to therapy	*rt-PA*	*SK*	*P*
Less than 3 h			
ECSG	23/29 (79%)	20/35 (57%)	0.06
TIMI	11/13 (85%)	11/21 (52%)	0.06
Combined	34/42 (81%)	31/55 (55%)	< 0.01
3 to 6 h			
ECSG	20/32 (62%)	14/26 (54%)	0.51
TIMI	89/130 (69%)	50/125 (40%)	< 0.001
Combined	109/162 (67%)	64/151 (42%)	< 0.001
Overall combined	143/204 (70%)	95/207 (46%)	

Data from ref 48.

The relative efficacy for coronary thrombolysis of APSAC has been determined in controlled comparative trials with both intravenous streptokinase[22] and with intracoronary streptokinase[23]. Brochier *et al.*[22] determined angiographic patency at a mean of 105 min after administration of APSAC or intravenous streptokinase and found patency frequencies of 72% in 42 patients treated with APSAC and of 56% in 44 patients given intravenous streptokinase, a difference that was not statistically significant. Anderson *et al.*[23] measured reperfusion rates in patients with proven coronary artery occlusion treated with APSAC or intracoronary streptokinase. When the authors compared reperfusion with APSAC at 90 minutes and with intracoronary streptokinase at 60 minutes, the reperfusion rates were 51% and 60% respectively, a non significant difference. The cumulative rate of reperfusion with intracoronary streptokinase was however markedly higher than that with APSAC at any given time point after the onset of therapy. In aggregate these comparative studies suggest that the efficacy for coronary thrombolysis of intravenous APSAC is comparable or somewhat higher than that of intravenous streptokinase, but lower than that of intracoronary streptokinase.

In the recently reported PRIMI trial[70] in which intravenous rscu-PA (80 mg over 1 hour) was compared with intravenous streptokinase in a double blind protocol, a trend ($p = 0.15$) towards higher patency rates at 90 minutes was observed for rscu-PA (72%) as compared to streptokinase (64%).

Relative speed of reperfusion

The average time to reperfusion in patients with successful thrombolysis with intravenous streptokinase, rt-PA, or APSAC is approximately 45 minutes.[23,29,57,69] However, available data suggest that there is a linear relationship between the cumulative percentage of patients reperfused at any given time point and the time elapsed since the start of the infusion. Consequently, the speed of reperfusion is proportional to the relative efficacy of the thrombolytic agents. Since rt-PA has a 50% higher efficacy for coronary thrombolysis than streptokinase, it will have a comparably higher speed of reperfusion. The relative speed of reperfusion with APSAC is less clear to the extent that its efficacy relative to intravenous streptokinase is not yet adequately established. In the PRIMI trial[70], patency rates at 60 minutes were significantly higher ($p < 0.001$) with rscu-PA (71%) as compared to streptokinase (48%).

Reocclusion

Reocclusion following successful reperfusion has variably been estimated on the basis of recurrent ischemic pain, ECG changes, release of cardiac enzymes and coronary angiography. Furthermore, reocclusion has been determined at different times after thrombolytic therapy, either during the early hours, the first days or at the end of the hospital stay.

Comparable studies with rigorously defined endpoints to assess reocclusion are scarce. Some authors have reported the incidence of reocclusion as high as 30% or more both for streptokinase and for rt-PA, whereas most frequently reocclusion rates of around 15% have been reported for both agents.[71]

Two prospective studies with rt-PA have been carried out that specifically address the issue of reocclusion, using angiographic endpoints at 6–24 hours[52] or at 24–48 hours.[72] The frequency of reocclusion was 7% of 73 patients in the first study, although three additional patients out of 60 reoccluded subsequently during the hospital course.[52] In the second study[72], the angiographically documented reocclusion rate was only 5% in 78 patients. In the largest available study with APSAC, the angiographically documented reocclusion frequency, between 90 min and 24 hours after treatment, was 8% in a subgroup of one third of patients treated, which is however an underestimate due to the fact that about one third of the patients had undergone additional interventional procedures.[23] In the PRIMI trial,[70] reocclusion rates at 24–36 hours with both rscu-PA and streptokinase were low, but some selection may have occurred due to frequent coronary interventions. Thus, presently available data suggest that reocclusion occurs to a comparable extent with all thrombolytic agents.

Bleeding complications

Bleeding complications in association with thrombolytic therapy are most likely due to the combined actions of the thrombolytic agents on blood coagulation components, on the vessel wall and on the hemostatic plug. In addition, demographic characteristics of the patient and adjunctive anticoagulant or antiplatelet therapy may contribute to a bleeding tendency. Quantitative and qualitative evaluation of a bleeding tendency and of spontaneous bleeding from results of non-comparative studies is very difficult, especially in association with highly variable frequencies of invasive cardiovascular procedures. Consequently, bleeding complications can validly be compared only in randomized controlled trials. In the four comparative trials with streptokinase and rt-PA, the frequency of bleeding complications was comparable in two trials,[33,73] and less frequent in the rt-PA group than in the comparative streptokinase group in the other two trials.[45,74] Although available data from small randomized trials suggest a somewhat lower bleeding incidence with rt-PA as compared with streptokinase, the markedly higher fibrin-selectivity of rt-PA has not resulted in a proportional reduction of hemorrhagic complications.

The contribution to bleeding of adjunctive anticoagulant therapy with heparin, which has been demonstrated for thrombolytic therapy with streptokinase,[75] will need to be explored further in the combination with rt-PA. In this context, the finding that bleeding times do not consistently prolong in patients during rt-PA infusion (no significant prolongation in 60% of the patients) and that there is no significant correlation between bleeding times and reperfusion[76] might be relevant and indicative of some degree of selectivity of rt-PA for a thrombus relative to a hemostatic plug. No data are available on serial bleeding times following streptokinase therapy.

A major recent concern with the use of rt-PA has been the occurrence of intracerebral bleeding in association with the use of 150 mg of rt-PA combined with heparin, in 1.6% of 1014 patients.[21] This frequency was found to be lower (0.6 percent) in 1,452 patients of the TIMI trial with the use of 100 mg of rt-PA,[21] and to 0.4% in 3,768 patients treated with 80–120 mg up to the summer of 1987.[77] Nonetheless, the possibility of intracerebral bleeding due to thrombolytic therapy remains a concern.

In the comparative trials with APSAC and streptokinase bleeding complication rates were found to vary widely, depending on the nature of the study (invasive or non-invasive). In the largest comparative study of APSAC with intravenous streptokinase[22] the bleeding complication rate was similar, whereas in the invasive study of Anderson *et al.*[23] bleeding and blood loss was more pronounced in the APSAC group than in the intracoronary streptokinase group. In the PRIMI trial,[70] bleeding complications were less frequent with rscu-PA than with streptokinase.

Table 6 *Neurological event rate in hospital following thrombolytic therapy with streptokinase or rt-PA*

	Number of	*Adjunctive therapy*		*Neurological Event Rate*		
Study	*patients*	*Aspirin*	*Heparin*	*Definition*	*Group I*	*Group II*
A. *Streptokinase vs. placebo*					*Placebo*	*Streptokinase*
ISAM[12]	1,741	+	+	ICB	0/882	4/859
GISSI[10]	11,806	?	?	Stroke	54/5,852	63/5,860
				SK-CVA	–	(0.2%)
ISSI-2[13]	17,189	+/–	?	Stroke	75/8,381	66/8,377
				SK ICB	–	(0.1–0.2%)
Total					129/15,115	133/15,096
B. *rt-PA vs. placebo*					*Placebo*	*rt-PA*
Van de Werf[19]	721	+	+	CVA	2/366	7/355
				rt-PA ICB		(1.4%)
ASSET[20]	5,111	–	+(24hr)	CVA	25/2,493	28/2,512
Total					27/2,859	35/2,867
C. *Streptokinase vs. rt-PA*					*Sk*	*rt-PA*
ECSG[45]	129	+	+	CVA	1/64	0/65
TIMI-I[69]	316	+	+	ICB	0/159	0/157
White[73]	270	?	?	ICB	1**/135	1/135
PAIMS[74]	171	–	+	ICB	1/85	0/86
Total					2/443	1/442

** During retreatment with rt-PA after reinfarction, not included in total.

Evaluation of the relative risk of cerebral bleeding in association with thrombolytic therapy is most important, but it is unfortunately confounded by several intervening factors. Firstly, acute myocardial infarction, even in the absence of thrombolytic therapy, is associated with an incidence of cerebrovascular accidents that has been estimated to be approximately 1% in the recent large clinical trials with streptokinase and rt-PA.[10,13,20] Secondly, it is difficult to discriminate between hemorrhagic and thrombotic strokes without the use of CT scans. Thirdly, thrombolytic therapy may convert a thrombotic stroke into a cerebral hemorrhage, without necessarily worsening the clinical outcome. Finally, adjunctive therapy may cause an increase in intracranial bleeding above the intrinsic and unavoidable frequency associated with thrombolytic therapy or specific thrombolytic agents. Therefore, the definitive answer to the question of the relative frequency of intracerebral bleeding associated with the various thrombolytic agents will require careful comparative studies with very large numbers of patients. Table 6 summarizes the results of neurological events during hospital follow-up in the large placebo-controlled trials with streptokinase or rt-PA and in all available small comparative trials with streptokinase and rt-PA. Although some evidence for treatment induced cerebral bleeding has been observed, the frequency of neurological events is not significantly higher than in the control groups. Consequently, preliminary results of placebo-controlled trials do not suggest that, at the recommended doses, streptokinase (1.5 megaunits) or rt-PA (100 mg) will significantly increase the combined frequency of thrombotic and hemorrhagic cerebrovascular accidents in patients with acute myocardial infarction.

Reduction of mortality

Mortality reduction in placebo-controlled trials has now been demonstrated for streptokinase, rt-PA and APSAC (Table 1). Streptokinase reduces overall mortality at 14–30 days by an estimated 25%. However, in the individual trials, mortality rates in the control groups vary between 6.5 and 13% and reductions in early (2–4 weeks) mortality with streptokinase vary between 18 and 81%. Clearly, the large variability in mortality in the control groups and the impact of streptokinase thereon are influenced by patient selection, by adjunctive therapy including anticoagulant and antiplatelet drugs, and by mechanical coronary interventions. In this context, it is virtually impossible to compare the in-hospital mortalities of uncontrolled trials after rt-PA treatment in patients with acute myocardial infarction, which average around 6% in the more than 5000 patients included in published studies, with those of streptokinase which average about 10% in the several tens of thousands of patients, treated with streptokinase since the placebo control rates also differ markedly, presumably due to patient selection.[3] The in-hospital mortality rates of the two placebo-controlled rt-PA trials,[19,20] also do not provide definitive answers concerning the relative impact of streptokinase and rt-PA on mortality. Indeed, in the ASSET trial, in the absence of aspirin, patients treated with rt-PA within 3 hours from the onset of symptoms had a reduction in mortality of 25.7%, whereas in the corresponding subgroup of the ISIS-II trial, the reduction in mortality with streptokinase was 27.6%. However, in the trial of the European Cooperative Study Group,[19] in the presence of adjunctive therapy with aspirin (and heparin), the reduction in mortality in patients treated within 3 hours of the onset of symptoms was 82%, whereas in the corresponding subgroup of ISIS-II (aspirin but not heparin) it was 40.3%. Furthermore, in the ISAM-study, with a control group mortality and adjunctive therapy similar to that of the European Cooperative Study Group trial, streptokinase had a markedly lower impact on mortality. In aggregate, these studies show that valid conclusions on the impact of thrombolytic agents will be obtained only from results of careful prospective and large comparative trials, such as the ongoing GISSI-2 and the planned ISIS-3 trial. Similar reservations hold for the interpretation of results obtained with APSAC.

If the clinical benefit of thrombolytic therapy in patients with acute myocardial infarction is proportional to the efficacy for coronary thrombolysis, the size of randomized clinical trials required to establish differences between thrombolytic agents can be calculated. On the basis of controlled clinical trials of streptokinase versus placebo, in over 35,000 patients with acute myocardial infarction, the reduction in hospital mortality in the treatment group was found to be approximately 25%. A hypothetical thrombolytic agent with a 50% higher efficacy of coronary thrombolysis than streptokinase would thus be anticipated to reduce early mortality by 37.5%. Assuming a control mortality of 9% in the absence of thrombolytic therapy, the mortality with streptokinase treatment would be reduced to 6.75% and that with the hypothetical more potent agent to 5.6%. In order to establish such a difference with a statistical power of 0.8 and a significance level of 0.05, more than 10,000 patients would have to be entered into a randomized trial. These numbers illustrate the tremendous task to be undertaken in order to translate efficacy for coronary thrombolysis into the most relevant clinical endpoint, mortality.

Table 7 *Comparative studies of streptokinase and rt-PA in patients with acute myocardial infarction*

Study	*Patient number*	*Early mortality rate*	
		SK	*rt-PA*
ECSG[45]	129	3/64	3/64
TIMI-I[71]	316	14/159	12/157
White[75]	270	10/135	5/135
PAIMS[76]	171	7/85	4/86
		34/443	24/442

In the meantime, it might well be of interest to review the available data from the four small comparative trials with streptokinase and rt-PA, carried out to date,[45,69,73,74] which are summarized in Table 7. Cumulative in-hospital mortalities were 36/443 (8.1%) in patients randomized to streptokinase and 24/442 (5.4%) in patients allocated to rt-PA. It should however be stressed that these results are derived from small studies, albeit randomized, which were not prospectively designed for a mortality endpoint. However, they agree remarkably well with the values estimated on the basis of the hypothesis that the clinical outcome is primarily determined by the efficacy of the thrombolytic agent.

New trends in thrombolytic therapy

Thrombolytic therapy for acute myocardial infarction, in its present form, is based on the premise that dissolution of the fibrin component of a coronary thrombus is necessary and sufficient for recanalization. However, this approach, even with the most potent thrombolytic agents presently available, fails in approximately 25% of the patients. In addition, large doses are required and the treatment is associated with unpredictable bleeding and with recurrent post-treatment ischemic events. Therefore the quest for further improved thrombolytic agents or alternative therapeutic regimens continues.

Acute ischemic coronary syndromes occur nearly always in patients with atherosclerotic coronary artery disease and in association with plaque rupture[78,79] which triggers intraluminal thrombosis.[7] The composition of the intraluminal thrombus formed in association with the rupture of an atherosclerotic plaque is heterogeneous, consisting of platelet-rich material contiguous to the area of plaque rupture, and erythrocyte-rich material extending both proximally and distally. This suggests two alternative and potentially complementary targets for coronary thrombolysis: the erythrocyte-rich whole blood clot and the platelet-rich thrombus. While the potential and limitations of fibrinolytic agents for the dissolution of whole blood clots is well known, the potential of pharmacological dispersion of platelet clumps and platelet-rich thrombus has not been fully explored. Furthermore, the mechanism of bleeding and strategies to reduce it need to be elucidated.

Attempts to improve the fibrin-dissolving potency of fibrinolytic agents

Present research in this area is carried out along several lines. In addition to the studies described below, several groups reported *in vitro* data on synergism of thrombolytic agents, mutants of t-PA or scu-PA, and hybrids of t-PA and scu-PA at the Congress of the International Society on Thrombosis and Haemostasis, Brussels, Belgium, July 9–10, 1987, with abstracts published in *Thrombosis and Haemostasis*, Volume 58, No. 1, 1987 and at the International Congress on Fibrinolysis, Amsterdam, the Netherlands, June 28-July 1, 1988, with abstracts published in *Fibrinolysis*, Volume 2, Supplement 1, 1988.

Synergism

The intrinsic fibrin selectivity of t-PA and scu-PA is mediated by entirely different molecular mechanisms. It is therefore not unreasonable to expect that, if administered in combination, the effect on clot dissolution would be more than additive. Synergism, if significant, would also allow a reduction of the total dose while obtaining a therapeutic effect that is equal to that achieved with higher doses of either agent alone. As a result, the potential for hemostatic side effects may be significantly reduced. In an *in vitro* system, composed of a ^{125}I-fibrin-labeled plasma clot immersed in citrated plasma, t-PA, scu-PA, and urokinase in molar ratios between 4:1 and 1:4 did not display significant synergism.[80–82] *In vivo*, however, in a jugular vein thrombosis model in the rabbit, significant synergism between t-PA and scu-PA and between t-PA and urokinase for thrombolysis was observed.[83] When t-PA and scu-PA were infused in a molar ratio of approximately 1:3, the specific thrombolytic activity of the mixture was approximately threefold higher than was anticipated on the basis of additive effects of both agents. The synergistic effect of t-PA and urokinase was only of borderline significance. A synergistic effect of at least a factor of two between t-PA and scu-PA was also found on coronary arterial thrombolysis in dogs.[84]

Preliminary results in patients with acute myocardial infarction [85,86] suggest that t-PA acts synergistically with scu-PA and urokinase in humans as well. Indeed, combining t-PA and scu-PA at approximately one-fifth of their individual thrombolytic doses produced coronary artery reperfusion in patients with acute myocardial infarction without associated systemic fibrinogen breakdown. Although these results are still preliminary and need to be confirmed in larger studies, they are potentially of significant clinical importance. The synergistic effect of t-PA and urokinase on coronary reperfusion has, however, not been confirmed in a large-scale study, although the use of the combination was associated with a significant reduction of the frequency of reocclusion.[68]

Mutants of t-PA and scu-PA

We have attempted to produce mutants of t-PA and scu-PA with improved fibrin-selectivity with the use of recombinant DNA techniques.

Deletion of specific domains of the t-PA molecule has been achieved. One of these t-PA mutants, called t-PA-ΔFE3X, a truncated t-PA molecule without the finger-like and growth factor domains and without carbohydrate side chains, appears to have an extended half-life and a slower plasma clearance rate *in vivo* and has retained most of its thrombolytic potency.[87]

Since scu-PA has intrinsic albeit limited plasminogen activating potential, attempts were made using recombinant DNA technology to prevent its conversion to two-chain urokinase. Two new constructs were produced by replacement of the lysine at position 158 with either glycine or glutamic acid. The kinetics of plasminogen activation with these mutants have been reported.[88]

Although these mutants do activate plasminogen to plasmin, their catalytic efficiency is only about 10% of that of the natural form of scu-PA. A clear dose-response relationship was seen when such mutants were injected in rabbits with an experimental jugular vein thrombus.[89] However, the specific thrombolytic activity of these mutants *in vivo* is also reduced by several fold. Thus, engineering of the scu-PA molecule, in order to prevent its conversion from a one-chain to a two-chain molecule, has not yielded improved molecules for thrombolysis.

Chimers of t-PA and scu-PA

Another approach has been to construct chimeric (hybrid) molecules that contain domains of both the t-PA and scu-PA molecules. The resultant molecule might combine the fibrin-affinity of t-PA (which is responsible for its concentration at the clot surface) with both the enzymatic properties of scu-PA (which is responsible for its stability in plasma) and the fibrin selectivity of scu-PA. One such chimer consisting of amino acids Ser-1 through Thr-263 of t-PA, fused to amino acids Leu144 to Leu411 of scu-PA, has been studied in detail.[90] Although this chimer has a higher fibrin affinity than scu-PA, its affinity is not as high as that of intact t-PA. Studies of the chimer *in vivo* indicate that it has maintained most of the thrombolytic potential of scu-PA, but does not appear to be a superior agent for thrombolysis.[91] The chimeric approach remains however promising, because it might enable the development of an agent that has increased fibrin selectivity at a reduced dose.

Antibody-targeted thrombolytic therapy

Several alternatives to target the action of thrombolytic agents towards the thrombus with the use of fibrin-specific antibodies are presently being investigated.[92,93] These include chemical conjugates of fibrin-specific antibodies with thrombolytic agents or recombinant fusion proteins comprising a fibrin-specific antibody site and the B-chain of t-PA. Alternatively, chemical conjugates between a fibrin-specific and a t-PA-specific antibody, and biosynthetically produced heteroduplex antibodies that are both fibrin and t-PA-specific, could bind to fibrin and localize endogenous or exogenous t-PA. These conjugates display significantly enhanced clot-specific lysis *in vitro* and, in an animal model, *in vivo*.

We have recently constructed a conjugate of rscu-PA with a murine monoclonal antibody directed against human fibrin fragment D-dimer that had an 8-fold increased specific thrombolytic activity *in vitro*[94] and an 8-fold higher thrombolytic potency in a rabbit jugular vein thrombosis model.[95]

Attempts to interfere with platelet-rich thrombus

The role of platelet aggregation in the pathogenesis of intraluminal coronary arterial thrombosis in patients with acute cardiac ischemic syndromes appears firmly established as reviewed above. Indeed, pathological examination has consistently revealed platelet-rich zones contiguous with plaque rupture in patients with acute myocardial infarction, unstable angina and sudden ischemic death. In addition aspirin appears to be efficient in the primary and secondary prevention of ischemic coronary events.[96]

Platelet disaggregation

Although the mechanisms of platelet aggregation and pharmacological approaches to interfere with the process are well known,[97] no efficient means are available to disperse preformed platelet-rich thrombus. In a plasma milieu *in vitro*, concentrations of thrombolytic agents that will rapidly dissolve whole blood clots, are virtually inactive towards preformed platelet aggregates[98] unless the platelets are pretreated with aspirin. rt-PA disaggregates platelet clumps but only at very high concentrations,[98] an order of magnitude higher than those currently achievable by intravenous infusion. This suggested to us that platelet-rich regions of coronary clot might be more resistant to lysis than erythrocyte-rich zones and that predominance of platelet-rich zones would limit the efficacy of intravenous thrombolytic therapy. Consequently, one approach to increased efficacy and speed of coronary artery reperfusion might consist of the pharmacological dispersion of platelet-rich thrombus, in combination with fibrin-dissolving therapy. Alternatively, specific interference with platelet deposition during fibrinolysis might accelerate thrombolysis and prevent reocclusion.

At present three approaches towards platelet disaggregation appear feasible. The first consists of the use of high dose intracoronary administration of plasminogen activators capable of disaggregating platelets. However, the logistic restrictions to intracoronary administration preclude its widespread use. The second approach involves the use of combinations of plasminogen activators with potent antiplatelet agents.[99] Thus, the combination of plasminogen activators with the anti-platelet GPIIb/IIIa antibody in animal models has resulted in accelerated lysis and elimination of reocclusion at markedly reduced doses of the fibrinolytic agent. In a third approach the thrombolytic agent could be targeted to platelet aggregates by means of specific monoclonal antibodies.

Prevention of platelet aggregation

Platelet aggregation clearly contributes to and may be the primary mechanism of underlying reocclusion. This is supported by our findings that monoclonal antibodies against platelet GPIIb/IIIa efficiently abolish reocclusion in animal models with intensive thrombogenic stimulus.[100] Finally, preliminary studies have indicated that arterial occlusion by platelet-rich thrombus cannot be prevented by heparin, but that it is efficiently prevented by local infusion of a synthetic thrombin inhibitor.[101] These results confirm and extend recent observations with a synthetic chloromethyl ketone.[102]

Attempts to reduce the bleeding tendency

The observation that bleeding also occurs in association with fibrin-specific thrombolytic agents has led to the hypothesis that these agents cannot distinguish between the fibrin of a pathologic thrombus and that of a hemostatic plug.[2,3] However, in a recent study with rt-PA in 50 patients with acute myocardial infarction, resulting in coronary artery patency in 83%, serial template bleeding times remained normal throughout the infusion period in 60% of the patients, despite full heparin anticoagulation. No correlation was observed between the template bleeding time and success or failure or reperfusion of the occluded coronary artery.[76] These observations are indicative of significant discrimination between hemostatic plugs and occlusive thrombi. The residual hemorrhagic tendency associated with the use of rt-PA despite its fibrin-specificity might relate to its interference with platelets[98] or with the endothelial cells[103] which may mediate enhanced local activation of plasminogen. Consequently, mutants of rt-PA with reduced affinity for endothelial cells might be associated with a reduced bleeding tendency. Elimination of the structures in rt-PA responsible for the interaction with endothelial cells, while maintaining those mediating the fibrin-specific enzymatic properties, might be possible with the use of recombinant DNA technology.

Conclusions

The beneficial effect of thrombolytic therapy in acute ischemic coronary syndromes, and particularly in acute myocardial infarction is now well established. The limited efficacy and potentially life-threatening side effects of thrombolytic agents remain a major problem. The present limitations of thrombolytic therapy can be explained on the basis of the heterogeneity of coronary arterial thrombus, consisting of both erythrocyte-rich and platelet-rich zones, and knowledge of the mechanism of fibrin-dissolution and platelet disaggregation. This unified concept suggests alternative and complementary pharmacological approaches to coronary artery recanalization. Available evidence suggests that the efficacy of coronary thrombolysis may be augmented either by improvement of the potency and specificity of fibrin-dissolving agents, by dispersion of aggregated platelets or by a combination of both. An at least partial discrimination between a pathological occlusive thrombus and a physiological hemostatic plug has been achieved with rt-PA and may be accessible to further modification. Continued investigations along several new research lines will provide new insights and promote progress towards the development of the ideal thrombolytic therapy, characterized by maximized stable coronary arterial thrombolysis with minimized bleeding.

References

1. Collen D, Stump D C, Gold H K, Thrombolytic therapy. *Ann. Rev. Med. 39*, 1988, 405–423.
2. Marder V J, Sherry S, Thrombolytic therapy: current status (first of two parts). *N. Engl. J. Med. 318*, 1988, 1512–1520.
3. Marder V J, Sherry S, Thrombolytic therapy: current status (second of two parts). *N. Engl. J. Med. 318*, 1988, 1585–1595.
4. Collen D, Regulation and control of fibrinolysis. *Thromb. Haemost. 43*, 1980, 77–89.
5. Collen D, Molecular mechanisms and clinical applications of thrombolysis. *Les Cahiers de la Fondation Louis Jeantet de Médecine 1*, 1986, 41–54.
6. Bachmann F, Fibrinolysis. In *Thrombosis and Haemostasis 1987*. Verstraete M, Vermylen J, Lijnen R and Arnout J (eds), Leuven University Press, Leuven, Belgium, 1987; pp 227–265.
7. De Wood M A, Spores J, Notske R, *et al.*, Prevalence of total coronary occlusion during the early hours of transmural myocardial infarction. *N. Engl. J. Med. 303*, 1980, 897–902.
8. Rentrop K P, Thrombolytic therapy in patients with acute myocardial infarction. *Circulation 71*, 1985, 627–631.
9. Gruppo Italiano per lo studio della Streptochinasi nell'Infarto miocardico (GISSI). Effectiveness of intravenous thrombolytic treatment in acute myocardial infarction. *Lancet 1*, 1986, 397–402.
10. Rovelli F, De Vita C, Feruglio G A, *et al.*, GISSI trial: early results and late follow up. *J. Am. Coll. Cardiol. 10*, 1987, 33B-39B.
11. Simoons M L, van de Brand M, de Zwaan C, *et al.*, Improved survival after early thrombolysis in acute myocardial infarction. *Lancet 2*, 1985, 578–581.

12. The ISAM Study Group. A prospective trial of intravenous streptokinase in acute myocardial infarction (I.S.A.M.). Mortality, morbidity, and infarct size at 21 days. *N. Engl. J. Med. 314*, 1986, 1465–1471.
13. ISIS-2 (Second International Study of Infarct Survival) Collaborative Group. Randomized trial of intravenous streptokinase, oral aspirin, both, or neither among 17,187 cases of suspected acute myocardial infarction: ISIS-2. *Lancet 2*, 1988, 349–360.
14. Kennedy J W, Martin G V, Davis K B, *et al.*, The Western Washington intravenous streptokinase in acute myocardial infarction randomized trial. *Circulation 77*, 1988, 345–352.
15. White H D, Norris R M, Brown M A, *et al.*, Effect of intravenous streptokinase on left ventricular function and early survival after acute myocardial infarction. *N. Engl. J. Med. 317*, 1987, 850–855.
16. Collen D, Human tissue-type plasminogen activator: from the laboratory to the bedside. *Circulation 72*, 1985, 18–20.
17. Guerci A D, Gerstenblith G, Brinker J A, *et al.*, A randomized trial of intravenous tissue plasminogen activator for acute myocardial infarction with subsequent randomization to elective coronary angioplasty. *N. Engl. J. Med. 317*, 1987, 1613–1618.
18. O'Rourke M, Baron D, Keogh A, *et al.*, Limitation of myocardial infarction by early infusion of recombinant tissue-type plasminogen activator. *Circulation 77*, 1988, 1311–1315.
19. Van de Werf F, Arnold A E R, Intravenous tissue plasminogen activator and size of infarct, left ventricular function, and survival in acute myocardial infarction. *Br. Med. J. 297*, 1988, 1374-1379.
20. Wilcox R G, von der Lippe G, Olsson C G, Jenssen G, Skene A M, Hampton J R, Trial of tissue plasminogen activator (rt-PA) for mortality reduction in acute myocardial infarction: the Anglo-Scandinavian study of early thrombolysis (ASSET). *Lancet 2*, 1988, 525–530.
21. Braunwald E, Knatterud G L, Passamani E, Robertson T L, Solomon R, Update from the thrombolysis in myocardial infarction trial. *J. Am. Coll. Cardiol. 10*, 1987, 970.
22. Brochier M L, Quillet L, Kulbertus H, *et al.*, Intravenous APSAC versus intravenous streptokinase in evolving myocardial infarction. *Drugs 33*, (Supplement 3); 1987, 140–145.
23. Anderson J L, Rothbard R L, Hackworthy R A, *et al.*, Multicenter reperfusion trial of intravenous anisoylated plasminogen streptokinase activator complex (APSAC) in acute myocardial infarction: controlled comparison with intracoronary streptokinase. *J. Am. Coll. Cardiol. 11*, 1988, 1153–1163.
24. AIMS Trial Study Group. Effect of intravenous APSAC on mortality after acute myocardial infarction: preliminary report of a placebo-controlled clinical trial. *Lancet 1*, 1988, 545–549.
25. Sherry S, Appraisal of various thrombolytic agents in the treatment of acute myocardial infarction. *Am. J. Med. 83*, Supplement 2A, 1987, 31–46.
26. Rentrop K P, Feit F, Blanke H, *et al.*, Effects of intracoronary streptokinase and intracoronary nitroglycerin infusion on coronary angiographic patterns and mortality in patients with acute myocardial infarction. *N. Engl. J. Med. 311*, 1984, 1457–1463.
27. Neuhaus K L, Tebbe U, Sauer G, Rahlf G, Kreuzer H, Kostering H, Hochdosierte intravenose Kurzinfusion von Streptokinase beim acuten Myocardinfarkt. In *Fibrinolytische Therapie*, Trübestein G and Etzel F, (eds), F K Schatttauer Verlag Stuttgart/New York 1983, pp 475–480.
28. Schröder R, Biamino G, von Leitner E R, *et al.*, Intravenous short-term infusion of streptokinase in acute myocardial infarction. *Circulation 67*, 1983, 536–548.

29. Rogers W J, Mantle J A, Hood W P, *et al.*, Prospective randomized trial of intravenous and intracoronary streptokinase in acute myocardial infarction. *Circulation 68*, 1983, 1051–1061.
30. Alderman E L, Jutzy K R, Berte L E, *et al.*, Randomized comparison of intravenous versus intracoronary streptokinase for myocardial infarction. *Am. J. Cardiol. 54*, 1984, 14–19.
31. Spann J F, Sherry S, Carabello B A, *et al.*, Coronary thrombolysis by intravenous streptokinase in acute myocardial infarction: acute and follow-up studies. *Am. J. Cardiol. 53*, 1984, 655–661.
32. Hillis L D, Borer J, Braunwald E, *et al.*, High dose intravenous streptokinase for acute myocardial infarction: preliminary results of a multicenter trial. *J. Am. Coll. Cardiol. 6*, 1985, 957–962.
33. The TIMI Study Group. Special Report. The thrombolysis in myocardial infarction (TIMI) trial. *N. Engl. J. Med. 312*, 1985, 932–936.
34. de Marneffe M, Van Thiel E, Ewalenko M, *et al.*, High-dose intravenous thrombolytic therapy in acute myocardial infarction: efficiency, tolerance, complications and influence on left ventricular performance. *Acta Cardiol. 40*, 1985, 183–198.
35. Collen D, Topol E J, Tiefenbrunn A J, *et al.*, Coronary thrombolysis with recombinant human tissue-type plasminogen activator: a prospective, randomized, placebo-controlled trial. *Circulation 70*, 1984, 1012–1017.
36. Williams D O, Borer J, Braunwald E, et al., Intravenous recombinant tissue-type plasminogen activator in patients with acute myocardial infarction: a report from the NHLBI thrombolysis in myocardial infarction trial. *Circulation 73*, 1986, 338–346.
37. Gold H K, Leinbach R C, Garabedian H D, *et al.*, Acute coronary reocclusion after thrombolysis with recombinant human tissue-type plasminogen activator: prevention by a maintenance infusion. *Circulation 73*, 1986, 347–352.
38. Mueller H S, Rao A K, Forman S A, *et al.*, Thrombolysis in myocardial infarction (TIMI): comparative studies of coronary reperfusion and systemic fibrinogenolysis with two forms of recombinant tissue-type plasminogen activator. *J. Am. Coll. Cardiol. 10*, 1987, 479–490.
39. Bonnier H J R M, Visser R F, Klomps H C, Hoffman H J M L, Comparison of intravenous anisoylated plasminogen streptokinase activator complex and intracoronary streptokinase in acute myocardial infarction. *Am. J. Cardiol. 62*, 1988, 25–30.
40. Dewilde P, Taeymans Y, Demoor D, Huyghens L, Block P, Intravenous thrombolysis with BRL 26921 in acute myocardial infarction. Presented at the International Symposium on Cardiovascular Pharmacotherapy, Geneva, 1985, Abstract 96.
41. Marder V J, Rothbard R L, Fitzpatrick P G, Francis C W, Rapid lysis of coronary artery thrombi with anisoylated plasminogen: streptokinase activator complex. *Ann. Intern. Med. 104*, 1986, 304–310.
42. Timmis A D, Griffin B, Crick J C P, Flax J S, Sowton E, An interim report of a double-blind placebo controlled recanalisation study of anisoylated plasminogen streptokinase activator complex in acute myocardial infarction. *Drugs 33* (Supplement 3), 1987, 146–150.
43. Taylor G J, Mikell F L, Moses H W, *et al.*, Intravenous versus intracoronary streptokinase therapy for acute myocardial infarction in community hospitals. *Am. J. Cardiol. 54*, 1984, 256–260.
44. Schwartz F, Hofmann M, Schuler G, von Olshausen K, Zimmermann R, Kübler W, Thrombolysis in acute myocardial infarction: effect of intravenous followed by intracoronary streptokinase application on estimates of infarct size. *Am. J. Cardiol. 53*,

1984, 1505–1510.
45. Verstraete M, Bernard R, Bory M, *et al.*, Randomised trial of intravenous recombinant tissue-type plasminogen activator versus intravenous streptokinase in acute myocardial infarction. *Lancet 1*, 1985, 842–847.
46. Cribier A, Berland J, Saoudi N, Redonnet M, Moore N, Letac B, Intracoronary streptokinase, OK! . . ., Intravenous streptokinase, first? *Haemostasis 16* (Supplement 3), 1986, 122–129.
47. Monnier P, Sigwart U, Vincent A, *et al.*, Anisoylated plasminogen streptokinase activator complex versus streptokinase in acute myocardial infarction: preliminary results of a randomised study. *Drugs 33*, (Supplement 3), 1987, 175–178.
48. Chesebro J, Knatterud G, Braunwald E, Thrombolytic therapy. *N. Engl. J. Med. 319*, 1988, 1544–1545.
49. Stack R S, O'Connor C M, Mark D B, *et al.*, Coronary perfusion during acute myocardial infarction with a combined therapy of coronary angioplasty and high-dose intravenous streptokinase. *Circulation 77*, 1988, 151–161.
50. López-Sendón J, Seabra-Gomes R, Martin Santos F, *et al.*, Intravenous anisoylated plasminogen streptokinase activator complex (APSAC) versus intravenous streptokinase (SK) in myocardial infarction (AMI). A randomized multicentre trial. *Eur. Heart. J. 9* (Supplement 1), 1988, 10.
51. Verstraete M, Bleifeld W, Brower R W, *et al.*, Double-blind randomised trial of intravenous tissue-type plasminogen activator versus placebo in acute myocardial infarction. *Lancet 2*, 1985, 965–969.
52. Verstraete M, Arnold A E R, Brower R W, *et al.*, Acute coronary thrombolysis with recombinant human tissue-type plasminogen activator: initial patency and influence of maintained infusion on reocclusion rate. *Am. J. Cardiol. 60*, 1987, 231–237.
53. Topol E J, Morris D C, Smalling R W, *et al.*, A multicenter, randomized, placebo-controlled trial of a new form of intravenous recombinant tissue-type plasminogen activator (Activase) in acute myocardial infarction. *J. Am. Coll. Cardiol. 9*, 1987, 1205–1213.
54. Topol E J, Califf R M, George B S, *et al.*, A randomized trial of immediate versus delayed elective angioplasty after intravenous tissue plasminogen activator in acute myocardial infarction. *N. Engl. J. Med. 317*, 1987, 581–588.
55. Topol E J, Bates E R, Walton J A Jr, *et al.*, Community hospital administration of intravenous tissue plasminogen activator in acute myocardial infarction: improved timing, thrombolytic efficacy and ventricular function. *J. Am. Coll. Cardiol. 10*, 1987, 1173–1177.
56. Topol E J, George B S, Kereiakes D J, *et al.*, A multicenter, randomized, controlled trial of intravenous tissue plasminogen activator and early intravenous heparin in acute myocardial infarction. *J. Am. Coll. Cardiol. 11*, 1988, 232A.
57. Simoons M L, Arnold A E R, Betriu A, *et al.*, Thrombolysis with tissue plasminogen activator in acute myocardial infarction: no additional benefit from immediate percutaneous coronary angioplasty. *Lancet 1*, 1988, 197–203.
58. Johns J A, Gold H K, Leinbach R C, *et al.*, Prevention of coronary artery reocclusion and reduction in late coronary artery stenosis after thrombolytic therapy in patients with acute myocardial infarction. A randomized study of maintenance infusion of recombinant human tissue-type plasminogen activator. *Circulation 78*, 1988, 546–556.
59. The TIMI Research Group. Immediate vs delayed catheterization and angioplasty following thrombolytic therapy for acute myocardial infarction. TIMI IIA results. *J. Am.*

Med. Assoc. 260, 1988, 2849–2858.
60. McNeill A J, Shannon J S, Cunningham S R, *et al.*, A randomised dose ranging study of recombinant tissue plasminogen activator in acute myocardial infarction. *Br. Med. J. 296*, 1988, 1768–1771.
61. Neuhaus K L, Tebbe U, Gottwik M, *et al.*, Intravenöse Infusion von recombinant tissue plasminogen activator (rt-PA) and Urokinase beim akuten Myokardinfarkt: Zwischenergebnisse der G.A.U.S.-Studie (German Activator Urokinase Study). *Klin. Wschr. 66*, (Suppl. XII) 1988, 102–108.
62. Neuhaus K L, Feuerer W, Tebbe U, Jeep-Tebbe S, Vogt A, Efficacy of a 90-minute infusion of 100 mg tissue plasminogen activator (rt-PA) in acute myocardial infarction. *Eur. Heart J. 9* (Supplement 1), 1988, 9.
63. Kasper W, Meinertz T, Wollschlaeger H, *et al.*, Coronary thrombolysis during acute myocardial infarction by intravenous BRL 26921, a new anisoylated plasminogen streptokinase activator complex. *Am. J. Cardiol. 58*, 1986, 418–421.
64. Monassier J P, Brochier M, Charbonnier B, *et al.*, EMINASE versus streptokinase à la phase aiguë de l'infarctus du myocarde: étude randomisée (étude I.R.S. II). 14e Congrès de Cardiologie de langue française; 1987, 25–30.
65. Relik-Van Wely L, van der Pol J M J, Visser R F, *et al.*, A preliminary report, on the angiographic assessed patency and reocclusion in patients treated with APSAC for acute myocardial infarction (AMI). A Dutch Multicentre Study. *Eur. Heart J. 9* (Supplement A), 1988, 8.
66. Vogt P, Schaller M D, Monnier P, *et al.*, Systemic thrombolysis in acute myocardial infarction: bolus injection of APSAC versus infusion of streptokinase. *Eur. Heart J. 9* (Supplement 1), 1988, 213.
67. Mathey D G, Schofer J, Sheehan F H, Becher H, Tilsner V, Dodge H T, Intravenous urokinase in acute myocardial infarction. *Am. J. Cardiol. 55*, 1985, 878–882.
68. Topol E J, Califf R M, George B S, *et al.*, Coronary arterial thrombolysis with combined infusion of recombinant tissue-type plasminogen activation and urokinase in acute myocardial infarction. *Circulation 77*, 1988, 1100–1107.
69. Chesebro J H, Knatterud G, Roberts R, *et al.*, Thrombolysis in myocardial infarction (TIMI) trial. Phase I: a comparison between intravenous tissue plasminogen activator and intravenous streptokinase. *Circulation 76*, 1987, 142–154.
70. PRIMI Trial Study Group. Randomised double-blind trial of recombinant pro-urokinase against streptokinase in acute myocardial infarction. *Lancet 1*, 1989, 863–868.
71. Raynaud P L, Desveaux B, Rëocclusion après traitement par l'Actilyse. *Arch. Mal. Coeur 81* (Supplement 1), 1988, 25–32.
72. Kent R S, Batson A G, LittleJohn J K, Thrombolytic effect of tissue-type plasminogen activator. In *Controversies in Thrombolysis*, Sherry S, Schröder R, Kluft C, Six A J, Mettinger K L (eds), Current Medical Literature Ltd, London, 1989, 3–14.
73. White H D, Rivers J T, Norris R M, *et al.*, Is rt-PA or streptokinase superior for preservation of left ventricular function after myocardial infarction? *Circulation* Suppl. II, 1988, II-303 .
74. Magnani B, for the Plasminogen Activator Italian Multicenter Study (PAIMS) investigators. Comparison of intravenous recombinant single chain human tissue-type plasminogen activator (rt-PA) with intravenous streptokinase in acute myocardial infarction. *J. Am. Coll. Cardiol. 13*, 1989, 19–26.
75. Schulman S, Lockner D, Granqvist S, Bratt G, Paul C, Nyman D, A comparative randomized trial of low-dose versus high-dose streptokinase in deep vein thrombosis of the thigh. *Thromb Haemost. 51*, 1984, 261–265.

76. Gimple L W, Gold H K, Leinbach R C, *et al.*, Bleeding time measurement predicts spontaneous bleeding during thrombolysis with recombinant tissue-type plasminogen activator (rt-PA). *J. Am. Coll. Cardiol. 11*, 1988, 231A.
77. FDA Summary Basis for Approval of Alteplase (86–0236). 1987, p 15.
78. Friedman M, The coronary thrombus. Its origin and fate. *Human Pathol. 2*, 1971, 81–128.
79. Davies M J, Thomas A C, Plaque fissuring – the cause of acute myocardial infarction, sudden ischaemic death, and crescendo angina. *Br. Heart J. 53*, 1985, 363–373.
80. Lijnen H R, Zamarron C, Blaber M, Winkler M E, Collen D, Activation of plasminogen by pro-urokinase. I. Mechanism. *J. Biol. Chem. 261*, 1986, 1253–1258.
81. Collen D, De Cock F, Demarsin E, Lijnen H R, Stump DC, Absence of synergism between tissue-type plasminogen activator (t-PA), single chain urokinase-type plasminogen activator (scu-PA) and urokinase on clot lysis in a plasma milieu *in vitro*. *Thromb. Haemost. 56*, 1986, 35–39.
82. Gurewich V, Pannell R, Synergism of tissue-type plasminogen activator (t-PA) and single-chain urokinase-type plasminogen activator (scu-PA) on clot lysis *in vitro* and a mechanism for this effect. *Thromb. Haemost. 57*, 1987, 372.
83. Collen D, Stassen J M, Stump D C, Verstraete M, Synergism of thrombolytic agents *in vivo*. *Circulation 74*, 1986, 838–842.
84. Ziskind A A, Gold H K, Yasuda T, Kanke M, Guerrero J L, *et al.*, Coronary thrombolysis in dogs with synergistic combinations of human tissue-type plasminogen activator (t-PA) and single urokinase-type plasminogen activator (scu-PA). *Clin. Res. 35*, 1987, 337A.
85. Collen D, Stump D C, Van de Werf F, Coronary thrombolysis in patients with acute myocardial infarction by intravenous infusion of synergic thrombolytic agents. *Am. Heart J. 112*, 1986, 1083–1084.
86. Collen D, Van de Werf F, Coronary arterial thrombolysis with low-dose synergistic combinations of recombinant tissue-type plasminogen activator (rt-PA) and recombinant single-chain urokinase-type plasminogen activator (rscu-PA) for acute myocardial infarction. *Am. J. Cardiol. 60*, 1987, 431–444.
87. Cambier P, van de Werf F, Larsen G R, Collen D, Pharmacokinetics and thrombolytic properties of a nonglycosylated mutant of human tissue-type plasminogen activator, lacking the finger and growth domains, in dogs with copper coil-induced coronary artery thrombosis. *J. Cardiovasc. Pharmacol. 11*, 1988, 468–472.
88. Nelles L, Lijnen H R, Collen D, Holmes W E, Characterization of recombinant human single chain urokinase-type plasminogen activator mutants produced by site-specific mutagenesis of lysine 158. *J. Biol. Chem. 262*, 1987, 5682–5689.
89. Collen D, Mao J, Stassen J M, *et al.*, Thrombolytic properties of Lys158 mutants of recombinant single-chain urokinase-type plasminogen activator (scu-PA) in rabbits with jugular vein thrombosis. *J. Vasc. Med. Biol. 1*, 1989, 46–49.
90. Nelles L, Lijnen H R, Collen D, Homes W E, Characterization of a fusion protein consisting of amino acids 1 to 263 of tissue-type plasminogen activator and amino acids 144 to 411 of urokinase-type plasminogen activator. *J. Biol. Chem. 262*, 1987, 10855–10862.
91. Collen D. Stassen J M, Demarsin E, Kieckens L, Lijnen H R, Nelles L, Pharmacokinetics and thrombolytic properties of chimaeric plasminogen activators consisting of the NH_2-terminal region of human tissue-type plasminogen activator and the COOH-terminal region of human single chain urokinase-type plasminogen activator. *J. Vasc. Med. Biol. 1*, 1989, 234–240.

92. Haber E, Runge M, Bode C, *et al.*, Antibody targeted fibrinolysis. *Thromb. Haemost. 57*, 1987, 253.
93. Haber E, Quertermous T, Matsueda G R, Runge M S, Innovative approaches to plasminogen activator therapy. *Science 243*, 1989, 51–56.
94. Dewerchin M, Lijnen H R, Van Hoef B, De Cock F, Collen D, Biochemical properties of conjugates of urokinase-type plasminogen activator with a monoclonal antibody specific for crosslinked fibrin. *Eur. J. Biochem. 185*, 1989, 141–149.
95. Collen D, Dewerchin M, Stassen J M, Kieckens L, Lijnen H R, Thrombolytic and pharmacokinetic properties of conjugates of urokinase-type plasminogen activator with a monoclonal antibody specific for cross-linked fibrin. *Fibrinolysis 3*, 1989, 197–202.
96. Harker L A, Clinical trials evaluating platelet-modifying drugs in patients with atherosclerotic cardiovascular disease and thrombosis. *Circulation 73*, 1986, 206–223.
97. Fuster V, Badimon L, Badimon J, Adams P C, Turitto V, Chesebro J H, Drugs interfering with platelet functions: mechanisms and clinical relevance. In *Thrombosis and Haemostasis 1987*, Verstraete M, Vermylen J, Lijnen R, Arnout J (eds), Leuven University Press, 1987, pp 349–418.
98. Loscalzo J, Vaughan D E, Tissue plasminogen activator promotes platelet disaggregation in plasma. *J. Clin. Invest. 79*, 1987, 1749–1755.
99. Yasuda T, Gold H K, Leinbach R C, *et al.*, Tissue plasminogen activator (t-PA) resistant platelet-rich white thrombus (WT) and combination treatment of t-PA and antiplatelet antibody to GPIIb/IIIa receptor (7E3). *Circulation 78*, 1988, II-5.
100. Gold H K, Coller B S, Yasuda T, *et al.*, Rapid and sustained coronary artery recanalization with combined bolus injection of recombinant tissue-type plasminogen activator and monoclonal antiplatelet GPIIb/IIIa antibody in a canine preparation. *Circulation 77*, 1988, 670–677.
101. Jang I K, Ziskind A A, Gold H K, Leinbach R C, Fallon J T, Collen D, Prevention of arterial platelet occlusion by selective thrombin inhibition. *Circulation 78*, 1988, II-311.
102. Hanson S R, Harker L A, Interruption of acute platelet-dependent thrombosis by the synthetic antithrombin D-phenylalanyl-L-prolyl-L-arginyl chloromethyl ketone. *Proc. Natl. Acad. Sci. 85*, 1988, 3184–3188.
103. Hajjar K A, Hamel N M, Harpel P C, Nachman R L, Binding of tissue plasminogen activator to cultured human endothelial cells. *J. Clin. Invest. 80*, 1987, 1712–1719.

INDEX